# THIS BOOK INCLUDES

# FREE RESOURCES

## TO HELP YOU BEGIN YOUR HEALING JOURNEY TODAY

### USE THE QR CODE BELOW TO CLAIM YOURS.

### "Can This Help Me?" Self-Assessment

A simple quiz to help you understand if you're a good candidate for The Victory Method.

### Smart Questions to Ask Any Provider

Your guide to getting the answers you deserve.

### 21-Day Victory Start Email Series

Daily tips and encouragement sent right to your inbox.

Free Resources

**VictoryInMotion.com/RepairNotReplaceBook**

# REPAIR
## — NOT —
# REPLACE

## NATURAL JOINT RELIEF
## WITHOUT
## SURGERY OR PILLS

## THE VICTORY METHOD TO HEALING

# Marc Patrick Pietropaoli, MD
### Foreword by James R. Andrews, MD

Niche Press
Indianapolis, IN

**Repair NOT Replace**

Copyright © 2026 by Marc Patrick Pietropaoli, MD, FAAOS

**Knee Repair, NOT Knee Replacement®** is a registered trademark of Marc Pietropaoli. CDE™, Clarity Day™, Comprehensive Diagnostic Evaluation™, Motion IS Medicine™, Repair, NOT Replace™, The Victory Journey™, The Victory Method™, The Victory Method for Functional & Musculoskeletal Restoration™, Victory AI Open MRI™, Victory In Motion™, Victory Repair, NOT Replace™, V-Motion Fit™, V-Motion Laser™, V-Motion Regen™, and V-Motion Slim™ are trademarks of Marc Pietropaoli.

**DISCLAIMER**
The information in this book is provided for educational and informational purposes only. It is not intended as medical advice, diagnosis, or treatment. Every person's health situation is unique, and you should always consult your own physician or qualified healthcare professional before starting, stopping, or changing any treatment plan. The therapies and approaches discussed in this book may not be appropriate for everyone, and no guarantees of specific outcomes are made or implied.

**A NOTE ABOUT THE STORIES**
All of the case studies in this book are based on true stories and real people. Each person's story could easily fill an entire book, so, to keep this book from becoming the longest book ever written (if I had my way, that's probably what would have happened), the stories have been shortened, condensed, and combined to convey all of the points and information I wanted to share while still satisfying my expert story coach, editor, and publisher.

For permission to reprint portions of this content or bulk purchases, contact info@victoryinmotion.com or call 315-993-KNEE.

ISBN
Paperback: 978-1-970329-01-8
eBook: 978-1-970329-00-1

Published by Niche Press; NichePress.com
Indianapolis, IN

Library of Congress Control Number: 2025924172

The views expressed herein are solely those of the author and do not necessarily reflect the views of the publisher.

Printed in the United States of America

*I dedicate this book to my father, Patrick J. Pietropaoli, Esq.,
as well as my mother, Victoria; my siblings, Tina, Maribeth, Rob
and Becky; my extended family; and all the amazing healthcare
workers — especially Anthony P. Pietropaoli, MD — who were my
father's caregivers during a very difficult time in his and our lives.*

*If this book can save one person and one family from what we
went through, it will be worth it. May it add fire to the knee
repair movement and help a world of people.*

# CONTENTS

# FOREWORD

# BY JAMES R. ANDREWS, MD

Over the course of my 50-year career, I've had the privilege of training and mentoring more than 650 outstanding young physicians. But every so often, a surgeon comes along whose passion, dedication, and long-term vision truly set him apart. Dr. Marc Pietropaoli was one of those fellows.

When Marc came to Birmingham to train with us at the American Sports Medicine Institute, he arrived with not only a strong surgical foundation but also a deep curiosity and a willingness to ask the kinds of questions that push our entire field forward. I remember well his commitment to his patients and his eagerness to understand not just how to operate but, more importantly, when *not* to operate — a philosophy I have always believed separates good surgeons from great ones.

What impressed me most about Marc during his fellowship was his early interest in biologics and the emerging field we now call regenerative medicine. At that time, platelet-rich plasma (PRP), stem-cell-based therapies, healing-laser technologies, and advanced rehabilitation techniques were still in their infancy. Yet Marc understood even then that the future of orthopedics and musculoskeletal care would not be defined solely by how well we could replace joints, but by how well we could repair and preserve them.

Over the years, I've watched with pride as Marc built upon those early foundations and developed one of the most comprehensive, thoughtful, and patient-centered prevention and repair programs in the United States. His *Knee Repair, NOT Knee Replacement*® philosophy reflects a modern understanding of joint preservation — combining precision diagnostics, regenerative biology, functional rehabilitation, and whole-body wellness to help patients avoid the pain, risks, and limitations that often accompany joint replacement surgery.

This book represents decades of Marc's work — not only as a surgeon, but as a teacher, a student of the science, and an advocate for patients. Marc has always believed that we should exhaust every reasonable option before offering surgery, and that belief is reflected on every page of this book.

For those who suffer from knee or other joint pain, who have been told replacement is their only path forward, or who simply want to understand what the future of musculoskeletal care looks like, this book will provide clarity, direction, and hope. Marc has taken the foundational principles he learned during his fellowship and elevated them into a system that is helping thousands of patients reclaim their lives.

I'm proud of the work he has done, and I'm honored to contribute this foreword to his important book.

— **James R. Andrews, MD**
*Founder, Andrews Institute for Orthopaedics & Sports Medicine*
*Founder, American Sports Medicine Institute (ASMI)*
*Founder, Andrews Research & Education Foundation (AREF)*
*Founder, Andrews Medicine*

# WHO THIS BOOK IS FOR

This book is for anyone who has been told a joint replacement is their only option. For people who've heard their surgeon say, "Come back and see me when the pain is bad enough that you want knee replacement surgery."

It is for spouses, partners, daughters, sons, mothers, fathers, siblings, family members, and close friends of anyone who has been told there is no other option but joint replacement or surgery.

It is for people who think, *There must be some other way.*

I am here to let you know your options aren't limited to joint replacement surgery or suffering through a lifetime of pain. There is a third option: to Repair, NOT Replace.

Not only is my goal to teach you about your third option, but my bigger mission is also to end the need for knee replacements by 2043. $1 of every purchase of *Repair NOT Replace* goes toward my $1 vs. $1 million challenge through which I intend to raise $1 million, $1 at a time. By scanning the QR code below, you can join the crusade to make the world knee replacement free by '43 by donating $1 or $1 million.

$1 vs. $1,000,000 Challenge

## WHO THIS BOOK IS NOT FOR

I am a highly educated and experienced fellowship-trained sports medicine orthopedic surgeon and regenerative medicine expert who loves to ask questions and obtain hard data. This book is not for people like me in a professional capacity. Personally, yes, professionally, no.

If you are a healthcare provider and you are looking for the science, data, how-to materials, etc. regarding platelet-rich plasma (PRP), bone marrow aspirate concentrate (BMAC), photobiomodulation, genetic-based diet, physiology, deep dives into fitness, bioidentical hormone replacement therapy (BHRT), or peptides, etc., then this is not the book for you. Everything in this book is supported by scientific literature and data tracking, but it is not meant to be a textbook or regenerative medicine review.

However, if you are a healthcare provider and desire to treat your patients better and give them more choices to eliminate pain and increase their quality of life, keep reading.

# CHAPTER 1

# THE WAKE-UP CALL

Marcia stood at her kitchen window, hands wrapped around a mug of cooling tea. Outside, her husband of 43 years was hunched over what used to be their prize-winning garden and landscaping.

Bill had always been the kind of man who found joy in physical work. For 35 years, he'd worked as an environmental tech at a medical device manufacturing company — walking, climbing stairs, hauling equipment, and solving problems with a grin. His weekends were for adventure: kayaking the Finger Lakes, hiking trails, and tending to and landscaping the garden that had become the talk of the neighborhood.

But now? Every movement was slow, deliberate. He'd take a few steps, stop, rub his knee, take another step, wince, shift his weight, then rub the other knee. Then his shoulder would flare up. "I'm falling apart," Bill told Marcia.

This wasn't the Bill she knew.

"I was losing him," Marcia told me later. "Not just to the pain, but to what the pain was doing to him."

The garden had grown wild. The kayak gathered dust. And the man who once whistled while he worked spent his days in a recliner, ice packs strapped to both knees and the right shoulder that had never fully recovered from an operation performed by another surgeon.

One afternoon, Bill shuffled inside, breathing hard.

"Banged my foot on that damn stump again," he muttered, rubbing his knee as he lowered himself into his chair.

Marcia looked at Bill and saw what I've seen in so many families: His greatest pain wasn't physical, it was the loss of self, of identity, of the life he once knew.

That's when she called our office.

## THE SYSTEM IS FAILING YOU

For more than 30 years, I've been telling patients there's a better way to experience relief from joint pain than cutting out your joint and replacing it with metal, plastic, and cement.

Right now, it's estimated that between 800,000 and a million Americans undergo joint replacement surgery every year.[1] That's more than 3,000 people every single day being told their only choice is to have their joints sawed out and replaced with artificial parts.

However, research shows that joint replacement surgery isn't always necessary. A 2014 study by Dr. Daniel Riddle found that one-third of knee replacements are unnecessary. An Australian review by Dowsey, Gunn, and Choong estimated that roughly one-quarter of hip and knee replacements may be performed in patients for whom surgery is considered inappropriate. And a 2018 study published in the *Journal of the American Medical Association* revealed that unnecessary hip and knee replacements alone cost Americans $8.3 billion annually — a figure that's likely doubled by now.[2]

Even when knee replacement surgery is considered appropriate, approximately one in five patients reports persistent pain, stiffness, or dissatisfaction after the procedure.[3] That means about 200,000 people every year go through major surgery only to still face pain, limitation, or the need for revision surgery in the future.[4]

What really bothers me is that most of these people were never told there was any other choice. They were simply told surgery was their only option.

At Victory In Motion, home of Knee Repair, NOT Knee Replacement®, we've helped more than 90 percent of our members reduce pain and restore function without surgery, without general anesthesia, without months of painful recovery, and without the lifelong limitations of artificial joints. In 2022, we tracked our patient results and found 91 percent of our patients reached their personal goals through our programs. Today, we continue to track our outcomes through the nationally recognized DataBiologics registry, where our patients consistently report an average 94 percent satisfaction rate and success rates ranging from 82 percent to 95 percent.[5]

Let me share what I've learned in 27 years of orthopedics, sports medicine, and now regenerative medicine practice: there is another, better way. And you deserve to know exactly what that looks like.

## WHEN EVERYTHING CHANGED

Bill had been told his knees were bone-on-bone and surgery was the only option. But years ago, he'd gone through a shoulder surgery that left him worse, not better, and he was not interested in repeating the experience.

"The surgeon I'd trusted to fix my shoulder told me I had a rotator cuff tear," Bill told me. "But when they got in there, there was no tear. And afterward, my shoulder was still killing me."

Bill hadn't just lost faith in his surgeon, he'd lost trust in doctors in general, and in the whole medical system.

It was no surprise then that when Marcia finally booked an appointment for Bill to see me, he didn't want to come.

"I came because Marcia forced me to," he told me when he first sat down in my office, "not because I believe this will work."

Looking at Bill across my desk, I saw a man carrying more than pain. He was carrying disappointment and fear. Fear of another failed attempt. Fear of false hope.

So, I told him what I say to every new patient who walks through our doors: "We don't just mask your pain.

3

We take the time and effort to figure out the root cause. We repair what's wrong. Not only do we treat the root cause, but because you're a whole person, we treat your whole body, not just your joint. It's a *whole-istic approach*, so to speak."

Bill looked at Marcia. She didn't speak. She didn't need to.

Finally, he said, "All right. Let's see if you're telling the truth."

A few days later, Bill limped through our door for his regenerative treatment. Two hours after that, Bill walked out of our clinic on his own. No hospital stay. No general anesthesia. Just a few Band-Aids where we'd used his own healing cells to start repairing what was damaged in his knees and right shoulder.

The three days that followed Bill's regenerative treatment were a little rough — I won't lie to you about that. Recovery isn't magic. Healing takes work. He was sore. He was skeptical. He was, as Marcia put it, "grumpy."

But by day three, the change began. Marcia saw it first: Bill stood from his chair without groaning. He walked to the mailbox without his cane. They were small victories, but when you've been living in pain for as long as Bill had, small victories feel like miracles.

Two weeks later, Bill was back in his yard and garden. And a couple months later, he hit that same stump again — and laughed.

"Didn't feel a thing!" he shouted to Marcia. Then, louder, with a joy she hadn't heard in years: "I'm cured!"

Of course, he wasn't cured. He was healing. But at that moment, Bill believed something he had thought impossible. He believed he could get better without surgery.

Six months later, a card arrived at our office. Inside was a photo of Bill with a huge smile on his face standing next to a sign that said Neighborhood Garden of the Year.

But it was Marcia's note in the card that said it all: "It's not just his knees and shoulder. We're kayaking again. We're planning trips. He whistles in the morning. I got my husband back. And we got our lives back."

## THE TRUTH ABOUT YOUR OPTIONS

Maybe you're reading this because, like Bill, you've been told that surgery is your only option.

Maybe you're like Marcia, watching someone you love fade under the weight of pain and discouragement.

Or maybe you're tired of hearing, "Wait until it's bad enough."

Here's what I've seen in my practice: The only way to avoid knee or other joint replacement surgery and get lasting relief is by following a whole-body healing plan that treats more than just your joint.

That's the truth the system doesn't want you to hear. Because as of 2025, knee replacements are a $10–12 billion a year industry.[6] Because insurance companies dictate what they'll pay for. And because too many doctors have been trained to offer only one solution.

But there is another way. A better way.

## THE VICTORY METHOD

Over the past 34 years, I've helped more than 30,000 people transform their lives by addressing knee pain and joint health in ways that no one else in the world does. Through my Knee Repair, NOT Knee Replacement system and The Victory Method for Functional & Musculoskeletal Restoration, we're committed to helping people get back to the things they enjoy most, *without* suffering through never-ending joint pain.

The Victory Method is built on four pillars:

### Pillar 1: Precision Diagnostics

This first step includes a Comprehensive Diagnostic Evaluation (CDE) to find the root cause of your pain, including but not limited to digital x-rays, Victory AI Open MRI, live ultrasound, lab work, a comprehensive medical history, a physical exam, and a whole-body evaluation. The vast majority of the time, this is completed in one visit, and almost never requires more than two visits. This experience is what we call a Clarity Day.

## Pillar 2: Whole-Body Wellness Optimization

Knowing that your knee or injured body part does not exist in isolation, we first want to make sure we are doing everything we can to make your body as healthy as possible so you can overcome your pain and limitations. We call this V-Motion Slim, and it includes genetic-based nutrition to improve gut health and potential hormone optimization to reduce inflammation throughout your entire system.

## Pillar 3: Regenerative Medicine Therapy

This pillar includes V-Motion Regen, which relies on your body's healing mechanisms to support the repair of damaged tissues. To do this, we use stem cells and other cells that help the stem cells from your bone marrow; platelet-rich plasma (PRP), which functions like your body's fertilizer, V-Motion Laser therapy, and additional advanced technologies.

## Pillar 4: Movement Restoration Through Victory In Motion Fitness

Personalized programs designed to improve total-body fitness through strength and conditioning can help rebuild strength, improve and optimize body movement, and reduce the likelihood of future problems. Victory In Motion Fitness (V-Motion Fit) is not simply a set of generic exercises, but a personalized program designed for your physiology, your condition, and your goals.

The Victory Method is *not* experimental medicine; it's medicine returning to its roots by working *with* the body's natural healing ability instead of against it. It's a proven process that doesn't involve pills and their nasty side effects, artificial cortisone injections (which are scientifically shown to actually damage cartilage and worsen arthritis), artificially made joint fluid injections (that, at best, last six months on average, and don't treat the root cause of the pain), and "assembly line" physical therapy that doesn't treat the whole body.[7]

## WHAT YOU'LL DISCOVER

In the chapters ahead, I'll show you:

- Why "bone-on-bone" is just a falsely negative description that doesn't convey exactly what's happening in your joint or how it can be treated.
- How your body's healing and regenerative potential is far greater than you've been told.
- Why treating just the joint with metal, plastic, and cement is like painting over mold. The problem won't be solved, and the solution won't last forever.
- The detailed, step-by-step elements of The Victory Method, which has helped thousands avoid surgery.
- Real stories about real people who dramatically reduced or eliminated their pain, healed their underlying joint conditions, and got their lives back in ways they never thought possible.

You'll meet Wayne, the corrections officer who was told at age 43 that he needed a knee replacement, only to avoid surgery for another 23 years.

You'll discover why Diane, at 79, can now kneel during her yoga exercises — something that's almost always impossible with artificial knees.

You'll learn why Jean, with one replaced knee and one repaired knee, wishes she'd known about knee repair through The Victory Method first.

And most important of all, you'll discover your own path to healing.

I promise you this: If you're willing to explore a proven holistic approach that reduces or eliminates your pain and helps your body heal itself without invasive surgery, I will guide you through every step of that journey.

*If you're willing to explore a proven holistic approach that reduces or eliminates your pain and helps your body heal itself without invasive surgery, I will guide you through every step of that journey.*

Before I show you the full Victory Method though, there's something you need to understand. I didn't always believe this type of non-surgery healing was possible either. In fact, I spent the first years of my orthopedic training learning the exact opposite.

I was taught that replacement was the gold standard. That there was no way to truly repair a joint once arthritis had taken hold. And that there was no way to offer my patients an alternative to the long, painful, and risky experience of surgery.

The reason I believe so deeply in my work today is because I've stood on both sides of the surgical table.

And what I saw — in one unforgettable moment — changed everything.

So let me take you back to where it all began.

# CHAPTER 2

# THE MOMENT THAT CHANGED EVERYTHING

A high-pitched whine cut through the operating room like a dentist's drill on steroids. Then came the metallic thunk of a hammer hitting a chisel, followed by bone and cartilage fragments flying through the air like sawdust in a carpentry shop.

I was 24 years old, a third-year medical student at Syracuse Upstate Medical University standing in the corner of Operating Room 3. This was supposed to be my dream, the moment I'd been working toward since my Uncle John, the original Dr. Pietropaoli, first told me, "If you want to be a sports medicine doctor, you need to become an orthopedic surgeon."

But as I watched Dr. David Murray, one of the inventors of modern knee replacement surgery, methodically saw through the end of a human femur (thigh bone), something inside me recoiled.

*This seems barbaric,* I thought. *There has to be a better way.*

The patient on the table was someone's grandmother. She'd trusted us with her body, her mobility, and her future. Apparently, our best option was to cut out large chunks of her cartilage and bone and pound metal, plastic, and cement into what remained.

Dr. Murray's technique was flawless. His hands moved with the precision of a master craftsman. But I couldn't shake the feeling that we were missing something fundamental.

Then I remembered something the junior resident in training had told me just before entering the operating room. "Feel free to ask any questions you want," he'd said. "Remember, there's no such thing as a dumb question!"

I was nervous, so I hesitated at first. Suddenly I remembered what my mother had always told me growing up: "Don't be afraid to question anything."

Shaking, I reluctantly raised my hand.

That same junior resident did a doubletake when he saw my raised hand, but he stayed silent. The nurses gazed at me. The anesthesiologist's eyes widened. And the chief resident, whom Dr. Murray was mentoring, glared with even more disgust than the nurses. No one acknowledged me — at least, not out loud.

Then, Dr. Murray peered over his spectacles and said, "Yes, Marc, you have a question?"

"Dr. Murray," I said, my voice barely steady. "Is there any way to grow back cartilage? Can we ever cure arthritis? Is there a way to repair a knee instead of replacing it?"

The room went silent except for the beeping of monitors.

Before Dr. Murray could get a word out of his mouth, the chief resident pointed at me with disgust and shouted, "No! There's no way to grow back cartilage. There's no cure for arthritis. The only way to treat arthritis like this is with a knee replacement."

I felt about two inches tall. Here I was, a medical student who'd been in the OR for all of 30 minutes, questioning a technique that had been invented by the man standing ten feet away from me.

And at that moment, I realized there was indeed such a thing as a dumb question.

After the surgery, Dr. Murray found me in the hallway. I was terrified, certain I was about to get the lecture of a lifetime about knowing my place. Instead, he said, "Marc, that was a really good question. And no, right now there's no way to grow back cartilage or repair the knee instead of replacing it. This is the best we have. But maybe someday you'll join us and figure out a better way."

In that moment, standing in a sterile hospital hallway, something shifted inside me. I wasn't just going to join them as a fellow orthopedist; I was going to prove that chief resident wrong.

*Challenge accepted!* I thought.

That was 1991.

Since then, finding a better way to repair joints became my mission.

If you've been told your only option is surgery, you're hearing the same voice that chief resident used with me.

But what if that voice is wrong? What if there really *is* another way?

## DISCOVERING MY OWN SPORTS MEDICINE DISNEY WORLD

Because of what Dr. Murray did for me that day, I eventually joined his orthopedic surgery residency program at Syracuse Upstate Medical University, and he became one of the greatest mentors of my life.

My orthopedic residency taught me to be a skilled surgeon. We performed surgery after surgery after surgery — every day for five years. I learned the intricacies of the knee, shoulder, hip, ankle — all the joints in the human body. I learned the techniques of replacement; the precision required to rebuild what trauma and arthritis had destroyed. Dr. Murray's training was exceptional, and I came out of my residency knowing how to operate with the best of them.

But there was a gap in my education. We learned very little about *care* in the office and how to determine when someone actually needed surgery, or how to manage their recovery. The attitude was simple: They all do great. Which isn't always true.

Committed to expanding my skills and knowledge, I began a year-long orthopedic sports medicine fellowship at the American Sports Medicine Institute in Birmingham, Alabama (ASMI). Working under Dr. James Andrews, who is widely regarded as the greatest sports medicine physician of all time — the GOAT — I was exposed to the revolutionary power of non-operative treatment.

Dr. Andrews was the most sought-after sports medicine surgeon by professional, amateur, collegiate, and even high school athletes from all over the world, and his goal was always to get a patient better without surgery *before* deciding to operate on them. Like the late Dr. Lewis Yocum, former team physician of the Los Angeles Angels, once said, "Jimmy Andrews taught us more about when *not* to operate than when to operate."

Dr. Andrews was a surgeon who, with the help of his fellows and his amazingly skilled team, would perform 20 surgeries or more *a day.* But based on demand, he could have performed two or three times that many. He chose not to because he and his team understood something profound: *the body has an amazing ability to heal itself.*

Under his guidance, the amazing educational opportunities at ASMI, and a large number of guest speakers, including the late Dr. James Bradley, the former Pittsburgh Steelers team physician, I learned about platelet-rich plasma, or PRP. By using the concentrated healing growth factors that already exist in a patient's blood and injecting them where they're needed most, we were able to accelerate the healing process. My first introduction to regenerative medicine would eventually take me all the way to where I am now writing this book for you.

(By the way, don't worry that you're going to be bombarded with a lot of medical terminology and acronyms. There really aren't that many, and I'll explain them all in simple language as we go along.)

While at ASMI, I was also extremely fortunate to work with Dr. Kevin Wilk, DPT, the greatest Doctor of Physical Therapy and Rehabilitation ever. (Okay, I'll admit I'm a bit biased, but Dr. Andrews and Dr. Wilk are both widely regarded as GOATs by all in their fields.) Dr. Wilk taught me how laser therapy could reduce inflammation and energize cells without any side effects — a technique that now plays a vital role in modern regenerative medicine.

Thanks to the many certified athletic trainers and strength and conditioning experts at ASMI, I discovered how blood type-influenced diet — the precursor to DNA-based nutrition — could address the root causes of inflammation and joint breakdown. "We are what we eat," as my mother always told me.

Let's face it, some injuries and conditions will still eventually need surgery, but Dr. Wilk's physical therapy techniques were able to prevent about 80 percent of ASMI patients from needing invasive procedures and joint replacements. Elite professional athletes would fly in to see Dr. Andrews, convinced they needed operations, and eight out of 10 of them would leave without surgery because of Dr. Wilk's skill and efforts. These weren't just any athletes — these were people whose careers depended on peak performance.

I'll never forget my first week when one of the greatest golfers of all time, a winner of multiple major championships, came in with a shoulder issue.

I'd watched this man win many a golf tournament on TV, and here he was, alone in a room with me. Talk about terrified!

"Hello, I'm Dr. Marc Pietropaoli, I am one of Dr. Andrews's sports medicine fellows in training. I'm going to ask you a few questions, examine your shoulder and surrounding areas, and then present your case to Dr. Andrews so he can decide whether you may need rehab or surgery."

He pointed right at me and announced, "No! I need shoulder surgery. When is Dr. Andrews coming in?"

I assured him that Dr. Andrews would be in shortly, but as I carefully examined him, I knew he wouldn't need surgery, and that Dr. Wilk was the one who was going to make him better. However, I certainly couldn't tell him that. Dr. Andrews always told us fellows, "Don't be the one to make the *big statement*."

Eventually, Dr. Andrews came in, examined this trophy-winning professional, sent him downstairs to Dr. Wilk, and the rest was history. The golfer never did have surgery and went on to win several more tournaments after that.

As my fellowship progressed, I continued to witness the miraculous healing these amazing doctors were able to achieve. I felt like I had found my own personal sports medicine Disney World!

So, if advanced, innovative, holistic, minimally invasive, non-operative, and regenerative techniques can help elite athletes avoid surgery and return to the highest levels of competition, imagine what they can do for everyday people who just want to walk without pain?

Dr. Andrews always said, "We treat *everyone* like an elite athlete." It's a mindset that's the foundation of incredible patient results, and it's why I believe so strongly that your situation isn't hopeless.

## THE MEDICAL SYSTEM FIGHTS BACK

When I finally hung up my shingle and joined an orthopedic practice in Auburn, New York, I was excited to offer patients what I'd learned. On my very first day, I saw seven patients.

One of those patients was Wayne, a 43-year-old corrections officer with severe knee pain. Every other surgeon had told him he needed a knee replacement. But after evaluating him, I believed we could first try other approaches I'd learned at ASMI under Dr. Andrews.

"You're only 43," I told him. "If you get a knee replacement now, it's going to wear out. Given your age, in 10–20 years you'll need a second knee replacement. Revision surgery presents a much greater risk of complications, doesn't work as well as the first one, and doesn't last as long. Let's try some alternatives."

Wayne was skeptical but willing. And his wife, a recovery room nurse who'd seen the realities and complications of knee replacement surgery, was relieved that someone was finally offering a different path.

At the end of that first day, I felt like my new practice had started out well. But then I ran into my senior partner in the hallway. "So how was your first day?" he asked. "How many patients did you see?"

"Seven," I replied.

"And how many surgeries did you book?" he asked.

"One."

His reaction was swift and harsh. He stared at me like I'd grown a second head. "I would've booked six! You need to do what the insurance companies tell us to do. They won't approve laser therapy or PRP. They'll only approve surgery. If you don't follow their rules, they'll drop us, and we'll go out of business."

This was my introduction to a system that prioritizes insurance approval over patient care. A system where a doctor's success is measured by surgical volume, not by helping people *avoid* surgery.

I felt crushed. Here I was, fresh from the Disney World of sports medicine, where I'd learned so much about both non-operative and the latest, cutting-edge, minimally invasive, arthroscopic operative techniques, including an introduction to regenerative medicine. Now I was being told that innovation had no place in my everyday practice.

Discouraged but undaunted, Wayne's results kept me going. Using the techniques I'd learned at ASMI in Birmingham — holistic rehabilitation, anti-inflammatory approaches, and other non-operative techniques — we helped him avoid surgery for more than 20 years. Wayne didn't get his knee replacement until he retired at 66, not 43. We gave him more than two decades with his own knee, and that eventual knee replacement is likely to last him the rest of his life.

Maybe you've also been told, "Surgery is needed *now*." But Wayne's story proves that's not always true. And that was with 1998 techniques. Today, our capabilities are exponentially better. Does that sound amazing to you? Are you interested? Keep reading.

## BUILDING SOMETHING DIFFERENT

In 2001, I was able to leave that practice in Auburn, New York. I could no longer stay in a system that refused to evolve and was less interested in customer care and healing than in financial expediency. I wanted to build what I'd envisioned in Birmingham: a practice that offered patients the full spectrum of healing options.

I knew I had to start from scratch, so I founded Victory Sports Medicine & Orthopedics in beautiful Skaneateles, New York. I started off with a staff of five, including our physician assistant, a nurse, two receptionists, and an office manager. Our team eventually grew to almost 50, but it has always embodied one simple principle: treat patients the way you'd want to be treated. Actually, treat them *better* than you'd treat yourself.

We called our mission "One-Up the Golden Rule." Building our approach took years of investment and innovation. We added advanced physical therapy that actually addressed the whole body. We invested in regenerative treatments like MLS healing laser therapy, PRP, and bone marrow cell therapy. We brought in non-invasive diagnostic tools, like ultrasound and open MRI, that could see problems before they became surgical emergencies.

Most importantly, we added proactive and preventive programs, such as Sportsmetrics, that are scientifically shown to reduce the risk of serious knee injuries by 50–75 percent![8] If we can cut the risk of serious knee injuries by that much, we'll see much less arthritis in patients and contribute to the ultimate goal of ending the need for knee replacements. Imagine if we could make this book obsolete with prevention!

Each addition of a new regenerative therapy or preventive treatment faced the same resistance from insurance companies and other doctors. But our patients kept getting better.

Each time we added something new, people in the medical establishment said we were crazy. "Patients won't pay for treatments insurance doesn't cover," they'd declare. "Other doctors will think you're a quack!"

But our mission wasn't designed for other doctors or insurance companies. We were building for patients just like you, who deserved more and better options.

Then came 2020.

> *Each addition of a new regenerative therapy or preventive treatment faced the same resistance from insurance companies and other doctors. But our patients kept getting better.*

## THE CATALYST

COVID-19 changed everything. Hospitals shut down. Operating rooms closed. Elective surgeries, including knee replacements, which I was still performing at that time, were put on hold indefinitely. Suddenly, all those patients scheduled for surgery had no choice but to try alternatives.

They were desperate. "When will the operating rooms reopen?" patients would ask me. "My knee is killing me. I'll do anything."

"I don't know when surgeries will resume," I told them. "But remember all those treatments I mentioned before that you didn't want to try? We can try them now."

For many of these patients, this was the first time they'd ever been forced to consider non-surgical options. They'd been so conditioned to believe surgery was inevitable that they'd never really given alternatives a chance.

But desperation can be a powerful incentive. These were people who'd literally run out of other choices. This was the catalyst I'd been waiting for. I combined everything I'd developed over the years into one comprehensive system of individualized, personalized programs. The results were remarkable. Patients who'd been told they had no choice but to undergo surgery were getting better without it. They weren't just managing their pain; they were actually healing.

People who'd given up hope were discovering their bodies could still heal. Patients who thought they were "too old" or "too damaged" were proving otherwise. The pandemic had forced them to try something different — and that something different was working.

Finally, on March 9, 2021, the US Patent and Trademark Office approved our trademark: Knee Repair, NOT Knee Replacement®. Twenty-nine years after I asked that impossible question in the OR, my clinic was officially offering a different answer.

Victory Sports Medicine & Orthopedics had evolved over the years from being primarily a surgical practice to a practice that rarely needed to perform surgery on patients. So, I changed the name to Victory In Motion. After all, motion *is* medicine!

## THE VISION BECOMES REALITY

Today, Victory In Motion, home of Knee Repair, NOT Knee Replacement, has helped thousands of people avoid feeling like knee replacement surgery is their only option. Most of our members tell us they're moving better, functioning better, and experiencing far less pain as they progress through our programs, which is reflected in the following two graphs comparing our real-world results to outcomes reported at other regenerative medicine clinics.[9] No one else is doing exactly what we're doing, which is why our results stand out.

# FUNCTION SCORE TREND OF KNEE-BONE AND JOINT

Scores range from 0 to 100, with higher scores indicating better function.

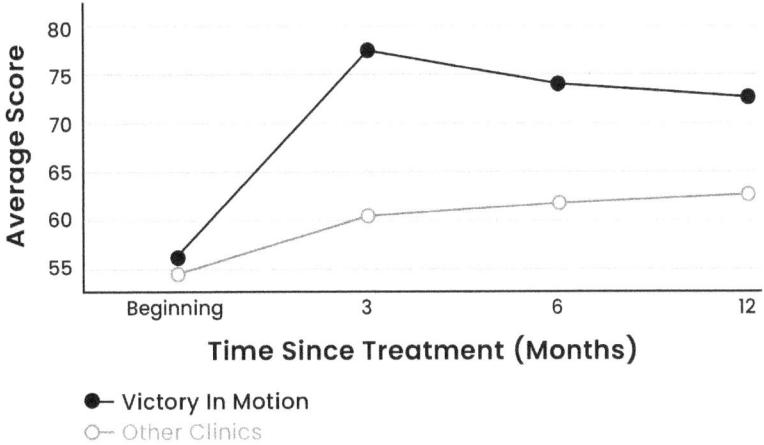

Time Since Treatment (Months)

●— Victory In Motion
○— Other Clinics

# PAIN SCORE TREND

Scores range from 0 to 10, with lower scores indicating less pain.

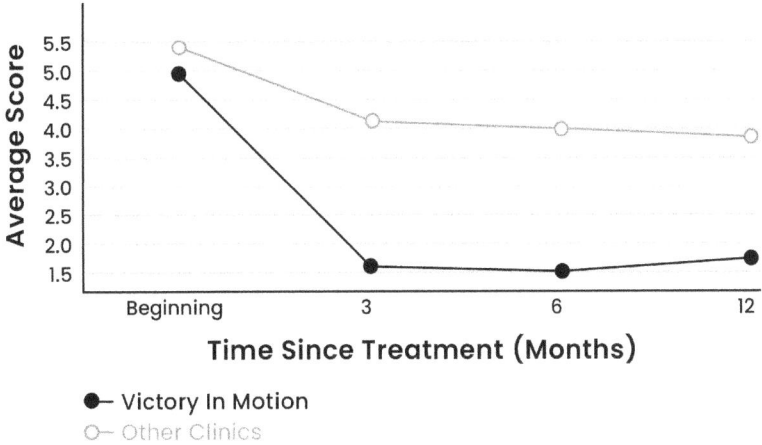

Time Since Treatment (Months)

●— Victory In Motion
○— Other Clinics

But focusing on regenerative therapies and preventive treatments isn't just about avoiding surgery. It's about addressing why joints fail in the first place.

In our current medical system, the old way treats your knee like a broken car part — remove and replace. The new way treats your knee as part of a living system that can heal when given the right support. The old way focuses only on the joint. The new way treats the whole person.

In the next chapter, I'll show you exactly how the old way and the new way compare in practice.

And you're about to discover exactly what that revolutionary new process looks like. Are you following this so far? Great, let's keep going.

# CHAPTER 3

# WHEN SURGERY ISN'T THE ONLY ANSWER

My father, Patrick Pietropaoli, was the son and grandson of Italian immigrants who taught him that in America, you could build whatever life you were willing to work for. He worked construction jobs to put himself through school, learning to use every tool in the box while earning his undergraduate and law degrees. Eventually, he became a respected attorney and, later, a judge.

He passed his love of building on to my brother and me. We didn't just learn to appreciate the physical act of creating something from nothing, but also the deeper truth that the right tools, used the right way, could fix almost anything. "Measure twice, cut once!" as he would say.

Golf wasn't just a game to my father; it was his sanctuary, his freedom, his way of connecting with the people he loved. Twice a year, he, with me as his partner, and my Uncle John, with my brother Rob as his partner, would face off at Oak Hill and Brook-Lea Country Clubs in Rochester, New York. These were affectionately known as "*The* Match" long before *The Match: Tiger vs. Phil* ever existed. My father and Uncle John talked about these matches all winter long. My brother and I enjoyed watching them argue and compete against each other just as much as we enjoyed playing with our family on such great golf courses.

But years of physical labor and an old water-skiing injury had taken their toll on my father. By the time I was establishing my practice, arthritis had begun creeping into his hips and knees. His shoulders were bothering him, as were his back and neck. He tried what the system offered: cortisone shots that gave him a few weeks of relief, gel injections that didn't work at all, and physical therapy that felt more like an assembly line than actual care.

Every time I tried to tell him about the amazing, non-operative techniques I was learning, my father always said, "My surgeon says my joints are bone-on-bone and I need a hip replacement, but I will probably eventually need both hips and both knees replaced. I just want to get it over with."

I was early in my career then, just beginning to explore alternatives like PRP and regenerative medicine. When I spoke to his surgeon, he shouted, "No!" before I could even explain the treatments I thought might help.

He said, "I've been doing this since before you were born, and there's no way to repair his hip. We have to replace it!"

It was like hearing that arrogant chief resident all over again, so I stopped advocating for a different treatment plan.

Looking back, my hesitation is one of my biggest regrets. I should have pushed back more on that old-school surgeon because, in the end, my father did what the system told him to do and he got the replacements.

## WHEN THE SYSTEM FAILS

The surgeries went well, as they say. He recovered. He could travel again, spend time with family, and even play golf. But anyone who knew him could see the difference in his personality. He could no longer do the construction projects he loved. His golf swing was restricted. His endurance was limited. The joy that used to radiate from him on the golf course had dimmed.

"At least I can still play," he'd say, and we'd all nod and pretend that was enough.

Nine years passed. Then came the phone call. It was Labor Day weekend, 2014. My brother, Rob — an internal medicine physician in Rochester — called with a tremor in his voice I'd never heard before.

"Marc... Dad's in the hospital. They think his hip is infected."

My stomach dropped. I knew what this meant. When you have metal, plastic, and cement in your body, no matter how far out you are from the surgery, bacteria can travel anywhere and set up camp. It's like they've found a fortress where antibiotics can't reach them.

The infection had taken hold deep in the artificial hip implant. They had to remove it, but even after several surgeries, the infection would not go away, and they had to leave the wound open to drain. It looked like a shark had taken a bite out of his outer, upper thigh. His care required multiple dressing changes every day, more surgeries, weeks of IV antibiotics, and months of antibiotics by mouth. My father, the man who'd built his life with his own hands, was now dependent on others for everything. Unsurprisingly, this took a toll on my mother, three sisters, brother, and the whole family, who were now acting as his caregivers.

When the infection finally cleared months later, his leg was five inches shorter. Five inches! The surgeons couldn't put an implant back into his hip because the infection risk was too high, so this proud, independent man now walked with a severe limp, his body twisted to compensate.

Sadly, my father's spirit never fully recovered. Within a year, he was diagnosed with pancreatic cancer. The doctors called it unfortunate timing, but I believe the severe ongoing stress, the chronic infection, the loss of independence — all of it contributed to his decline.

He tried once, but he never played a full round of golf again. His golf clubs gathered dust in the corner of his garage.

Standing in that hospital room, watching my father suffer from a "successful" surgery that had stolen everything he loved, I made a vow: I will never stay silent again. I will push back against the system.

I don't want another person and another family to go through what we had to go through. There *is* another way — and my patients and the world deserve to know about it.

> *Standing in that hospital room, watching my father suffer from a "successful" surgery that had stolen everything he loved, I made a vow: I will never stay silent again. I will push back against the system.*

## A DIFFERENT STORY

What if someone could experience both approaches to repairing or replacing joints and tell us which one actually works better?

I've had many patients who underwent knee replacement on one leg at another facility, then didn't want a knee replacement on the opposite leg because they didn't want to go through all of the pain, long recovery, large incision, and many risks again.

That is why I want you to meet Jean, who, at 82, valued her independence above everything else. "I don't want to run marathons," she'd tell me. "I just want to stay independent."

Unfortunately, her independence was slipping away one painful step at a time.

Years earlier, Jean had undergone a total knee replacement on her right leg. The surgery went fine — if you consider having huge hunks of cartilage and bone replaced by metal, plastic, and cement *fine* — but the recovery was "brutal," as Jean put it. Six weeks using a walker, months of physical therapy, and learning to live with permanent limitations hardly felt worth the reward.

"I can't kneel anymore," she explained. "There's a constant numbness and stiffness in the replacement knee. And that clicking sound when I walk? It's like I'm part robot. I swore I'd never do that again."

But then her left knee started failing. Simple tasks, like standing at the sink to wash dishes and climbing the stairs, became daily battles. With macular degeneration already affecting her balance, her legs were her lifeline. She couldn't afford to lose them.

Jean tried everything insurance would cover. Cortisone shots that barely touched the pain. Gel injections that did nothing. Physical therapy with the same generic exercises. Pain medications that made her foggy or upset her stomach. Nothing worked.

The breaking point came one afternoon when her husband, Dick, was sitting comfortably in his recliner and noticed the carpet needed attention.

"Honey, the floor's getting pretty dirty," he observed.

"Yeah, because my knee is killing me, and I can't vacuum. Maybe you can get off your fat ass and do it yourself!" she snapped, her usually joyful attitude slipping away.

That moment of frustration crystallized what she was really fighting for: not just pain relief, but her independence, her ability to take care of her home, and her dignity.

"You need another knee replacement," her surgeon announced, as if delivering a weather report.

Jean's response was immediate: "No."

That's when she heard about our Knee Repair, NOT Knee Replacement approach. She was skeptical but desperate. "Is this real?" she asked me during her consultation. "Could it really help me?"

"If you don't mind me geeking out a little," I said, "let me tell you about Dr. Philippe Hernigou, an orthopedic surgeon from France."

Then I told her about the study that transformed my approach to orthopedic medicine and cemented my Knee Repair, NOT Knee Replacement journey.

"Starting in 2000, Dr. Hernigou took 140 patients like you who had arthritis in both knees and performed a traditional replacement surgery on one of their knees. On the patient's *other* leg, he took bone marrow stem cells and injected them into the damaged soft bone in the non-replaced knee.

"Stem cells are cells that have not turned into anything yet and can turn into bone, tendon, cartilage, heart, kidney, lung, etc. in the right circumstances. Dr. Hernigou believed that the bone marrow cells from these patients could help the damaged, microfractured bone in their knees *actually heal* so those knees wouldn't need to be surgically removed and replaced.

"For the next ten to twenty years, he followed up with these patients to measure their progress. Miraculously, 82 percent of the knees that were given bone marrow stem cells didn't need to be replaced for at least ten years, and sometimes as many as twenty!"

As I finished telling Jean the story about Dr. Hernigou's work, I could see that her skeptical expression had been replaced by one of fascination and hope.

"Jean, you've been told you *have to* have surgery to replace your knee, correct?" I asked.

She nodded.

"Let me ask you this: If I told you that you have an 82 percent chance of living another ten to twenty years without having the hospital stay, risk, pain, and long recovery related to having your remaining knee surgically replaced, and instead experienced a few 'poke holes' and injections, what would you say?"

Jean raised her hand and said, without hesitation, "I'd say *sign me up*. When can we start?"

We scheduled the regenerative medicine injection portion of Jean's Victory Journey Program for the following Tuesday morning. But on the day of her treatment, disaster struck — a power outage shut down our facility.

"I was crushed," Jean told me later. "I'd finally gotten my mind ready for this. I'd psyched myself up. *Now what? I'd thought.*"

Fortunately, power was restored within hours, and her regenerative medicine procedure went forward as planned. And when it was over, Jean couldn't believe what had just happened.

"I walked out with just a Band-Aid on my knee," she recalls, still amazed years later. "No incision. No hospital stay. No walker. No narcotics. Just a Band-Aid! And I actually *walked* out that day! I hadn't been able to walk that well for at least six weeks after my knee replacement. I was truly amazed!"

## THE TRANSFORMATION

The real work of Jean's Victory Journey began after her initial platelet and bone marrow injection. Now it was time for her V-Motion Laser therapy to energize the mitochondria in the cells surrounding her knee.

You remember learning about mitochondria back in high school Biology class, right? It's the *powerhouse of the cell.* See? You do remember some science!

The healing laser also reduces inflammation and swelling, increases blood flow, and inhibits the painful nerve fibers, the nociceptors that cause pain. Because of this treatment, Jean did not have to take any addictive narcotics that made her unsteady on her feet.

Shortly after her laser treatment, she began our V-Motion Fit, total-body fitness, strength and conditioning program designed to help her whole body. "I even posed for a social media post doing kettlebell dead lifts with Adam, my V-Motion Fit specialist," she told me with a laugh.

Jean's progress was gradual — there were no overnight miracles — but much faster than her recovery had been after her knee replacement. She had less pain at the sink, more strength on stairs, and better balance overall.

Months later, Jean picked up the same vacuum that had sparked the heated exchange with her husband and noticed something remarkable.

"When I used to vacuum, my right knee, the replaced one, would kill me," she explained. "All that pivoting and pushing was too much, and I couldn't kneel to get under furniture. But now I can actually kneel down with my left knee when I need to. It's like having my real knee back."

Today, Jean lives with both approaches to joint repair in her body — a daily comparison study. Her right knee, the replaced one, remains functional, but stiff and numb. She still can't kneel on it. It still clicks when she walks. But it's considered "successful" by surgical standards.

Her left knee? It's almost pain-free. She can handle stairs, including the spiral staircase in her home. She does her own housework. Most importantly, she avoided that second devastating surgery she swore she'd never endure again.

"Don't blindly accept surgery as your only option," Jean tells anyone who'll listen. "Learn what else is available. You might not have to go through what I did the first time."

## THE REAL DIFFERENCE

Jean's story reveals the fundamental difference between the old way and the new way.

**The Old Way:** Treats your symptoms with mechanical, unnatural solutions. The plan is to remove the worn part, install artificial components, and hope for the best. Accept limitations and risks as inevitable.

**The New Way:** Treats you as a whole person with biological, natural solutions. Addresses why your joint failed, optimizes your body's healing environment, repairs what's damaged, and restores your natural function. Much less risky.

**The Old Way:** Relies on cortisone shots, pain pills, and generic physical therapy. Then you undergo surgery when those fail.

And here's something that should make you angry: several studies have shown that patients who received cortisone injections had **faster cartilage wear** compared to those who didn't get the shots.[10] Cortisone might reduce inflammation temporarily, but it actually damages the cartilage it's supposed to help, yet it's still the first thing most doctors reach for. It's not their fault though. They're just implementing the training we've all been given by the "system."

**The New Way:** Leverages genetic nutrition based on your own personal DNA. Precision diagnostics, regenerative therapy, bioidentical hormone therapy (BHRT), total-body fitness, strength and conditioning are all personalized and working together for you.

**The Old Way:** You have a slow recovery, permanent limitations, and require lifelong maintenance. There's also a lifelong risk of complications, infection, and the need for a new revision replacement years later.

**The New Way:** You have a faster recovery, restored function, lasting natural results, and minimal risk of infection.

Every time Jean vacuums her house now, she's reminded that the only solution she was told about wasn't the only one after all. But even with this knowledge, I know you might be convinced that your situation is different and *repairing* your joint wouldn't work for you. Maybe you believe you're too old, too damaged, or that you've already tried everything.

These aren't character flaws; they're human responses to disappointment and pain. In the next chapter, I want to address what's really holding you back from healing, because the biggest barrier to your recovery might not be your knee or whatever body part is ailing you at all, it might be the story you're telling yourself about what's possible.

> *The biggest barrier to your recovery might not be your knee or whatever body part is ailing you at all, it might be the story you're telling yourself about what's possible.*

# CHAPTER 4

# WHAT'S HOLDING YOU BACK?

By now you might be feeling one of two things: You're either starting to believe that maybe, just maybe, there really is another way, or you're hearing the voice in your head that's listing all the reasons why this won't work for you.

*I'm too old.*

*My damage is too far gone.*

*I've already tried everything.*

*My doctor said surgery is my only option.*

*This isn't the right time.*

Sound familiar? These aren't just excuses. They're real fears based on real experiences. Every single patient who's walked through our doors has experienced at least one of these fears or false beliefs — including me. And I'm supposed to be the expert who knows better.

## THE DOCTOR BECOMES THE PATIENT

I was cooking a Mother's Day dinner for my wife and family, trying to show what a good husband and father I was by making my famous Italian red sauce from the tomatoes I'd grown in my garden.

Then, somehow, I tweaked my elbow while chopping up garlic and onions with a slicer-dicer. The pain shot through my arm, but I did what most of us do and told myself it was nothing.

Except, it wasn't nothing.

Over the years, that elbow pain became my constant companion. I tried everything I'd normally recommend: physical therapy, anti-inflammatory medications, compression straps, and even laser therapy by itself.

They helped temporarily but never fixed the real underlying root problem. So, I learned to work around it, adjusting how I operated, how I examined patients, how I shook hands at Mass, and pretty much how I managed to do everything with my right arm and hand.

I kept telling myself the same lie my patients tell themselves: "I can manage it. I don't have time to deal with this right now."

Then came Father's Day, 2023. My family, knowing my love of cooking, gifted me an Ooni pizza oven. If you've never used one, they're incredible. You can make restaurant-quality, wood-fired pizza in your own backyard. They're also blazing hot, requiring you to constantly turn the pizzas with quick, repetitive motions.

Two weeks later, I got carried away. I made 23 pizzas in one hour for our Independence Day party. By pizza number 15, I knew I was in trouble. By number 23, I could barely lift my arm.

The MRI I got a few days later confirmed what I'd feared: my tendon was hanging by a thread. One wrong move and it would tear completely, requiring surgery that would sideline me from work for months.

I found myself sitting in my office, staring at those MRI images, thinking exactly what my patients think: *Maybe I can get by a while longer.* After all, we had a long-planned family trip to my wife's native Portugal coming up.

Then, just prior to leaving for that trip, I found out I was going to be a grandfather, and my granddaughter was due in April of the following year. It was one of the greatest days of my life.

When we got back from Portugal, I made it my goal to thoroughly train Jordan, my physician assistant, on the entire Knee Repair, NOT Knee Replacement program. It was especially important for him to learn how to harvest the bone marrow cells that contain stem cells and other helper cells, prepare the PRP, and inject it into whatever body part needs healing. I knew it would take several months of intense training, but Jordan was up to the task.

By the time I got Jordan fully trained, it was getting close to my granddaughter's due date.

I'd been doing a lot of strengthening exercises and even some handheld laser therapy on my elbow and it was feeling better but wasn't 100 percent. I knew I needed to do something more to repair my tendon, but I started to rationalize and make excuses to try and give myself an out. Sound familiar?

When my wife, Cristina, saw me constantly rubbing my elbow, she declared, "You need to do something about that!"

"I know," I answered meekly. "But I'm starting to think this isn't the right time. Baby Lyla is due in a couple of weeks, and I want to be able to hold her after she's born. Plus, I've got procedures and surgeries scheduled, patients who need me, and the practice is busier than ever..."

She cut me off with five short words: "There's never a perfect time."

Then she hit me with a truth that only someone who loves you can deliver. "Lyla won't remember you not holding her now because your elbow hurts. But she *will* remember if you can't throw a ball to her when she's five because you were too stubborn to fix it now."

She was right. I was doing exactly what I tell my patients not to do by letting fear disguise itself as the misguided belief that waiting for the perfect moment was the responsible choice.

The next week, I scheduled my procedure with Jordan. The irony wasn't lost on me — I'd spent months teaching him these procedures, and now I'd be on the receiving end.

> *I was doing exactly what I tell my patients not to do by letting fear disguise itself as the misguided belief that waiting for the perfect moment was the responsible choice.*

"You know," I told Jordan as I lay on the exam table in nothing but paper shorts, prepping for the bone marrow stem cell harvest, "filming this for educational purposes seemed like a much better idea when it wasn't my butt on camera."

But beyond the humor was a deeper realization: This is what my patients feel. This vulnerability. This hope mixed with doubt. This fear that maybe nothing will work.

I wasn't the doctor anymore. I was the patient. Scared and hoping this would work.

## The First 72 Hours

I won't lie to you, the first night was rough. My elbow throbbed. The swelling made it difficult to find a comfortable position, but it wasn't nearly as painful as the five different surgeries I'd had in the past.

Fractured cheekbone with plate and screws? Painful.

Torn knee meniscus cartilage surgery? Painful.

Vasectomy? Okay, not that painful, physically. But mentally? Painful.

Mass removal? Painful.

Umbilical hernia repair? Very painful.

Still, I lay in bed at 3:00 a.m. thinking, *What if this doesn't work?*

This was my own medicine, my own treatment protocol. I knew the science behind *why* and *how* our program worked to repair joints, muscles, ligaments, and tendons. I knew the healing cascade typically begins within 24–48 hours after treatment as growth factors from platelets start signaling repair. I knew the stem cells and other regenerative cells begin differentiating and proliferating around day three to seven.[11] But when it's your body, when you're the one lying there in pain, doubt can creep in differently.

"I expected this," I reminded myself. "I tell patients to expect this. The inflammation is part of the normal, early healing process and is actually a *good* thing. It means my body is responding to the treatment."

But knowing something intellectually and experiencing it physically are two different things. By morning, I was tired and upset at myself for second-guessing everything. I was *very* excited to get going and get started!

The second night was somewhat better. The throbbing had shifted to a dull ache. By the third night, I was ready to start the next phase and begin V-Motion Fit.

## Your Personal Tour Guide

V-Motion Fit is the holistic program focusing on total-body fitness, strength, and conditioning that I developed in 2011, and it's an integral part of Knee Repair, NOT Knee Replacement and The Victory Journey. Unlike cookie-cutter workouts or standard physical therapy, V-Motion Fit addresses the whole person, tailoring each program to individual needs and goals. It's personalized, supervised, and medically guided — the vital part of the program where movement becomes medicine.

Our V-Motion Fit specialists are like holistic tour guides for your health journey. They take your hand and literally guide you through the system of total-body fitness and strength and conditioning and map your safest, most effective path back to strength, freedom, and attaining the goals and dreams you desire. Instead of treating just the knee or other injured body part, your V-Motion Fit certified guide helps restore the whole person, ensuring long-term results.

## V-MOTION FIT™ TOUR GUIDE

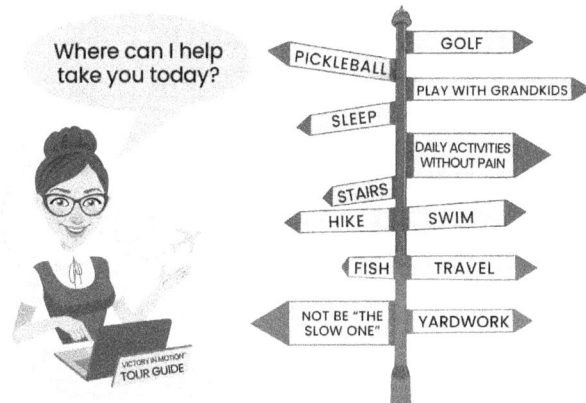

Where can I help take you today?

GOLF
PICKLEBALL
PLAY WITH GRANDKIDS
SLEEP
DAILY ACTIVITIES WITHOUT PAIN
STAIRS
HIKE
SWIM
FISH
TRAVEL
NOT BE "THE SLOW ONE"
YARDWORK

VICTORY IN MOTION
TOUR GUIDE

Two days after starting V-Motion Fit, I was back doing my job as a surgeon in the operating room, performing arthroscopic surgeries, which don't require heavy lifting.

In the end, I never missed a single day of work!

And throughout my entire recovery, I was able to keep working. Not because I'm some kind of hero, but because I needed to prove to myself what I tell my patients: Motion IS Medicine. You can heal while living your life.

> *Motion IS Medicine.*

## The Overconfidence Trap

By the second week of my twelve-week V-Motion Fit program, I felt fantastic. The combination of V-Motion Fit training and MLS laser therapy was working even better than expected. My range of motion had returned to normal, and my pain was almost non-existent.

That's when I made the classic mistake I caution all my patients to avoid. I got cocky.

I started lifting heavier weights than prescribed, doing more reps than recommended, and testing my patients' strength and stability a little too vigorously while performing physical exams.

And then there was the garden.

My father-in-law, 95 years old at the time, Portuguese, and hard of hearing, had been watching me neglect our vegetable gardens as I worked on healing my elbow. One afternoon, he cornered me with the subtlety of a sledgehammer.

"Dr. Marc!" he shouted, pointing at the overgrown tomatoes. "You no do nothing in the garden. I farmer. You not a farmer!"

We have a friendly gardening rivalry, so his words spurred me into action. There I was, little more than two weeks post-procedure, wrestling with tomato stakes and hauling bags of topsoil because I couldn't admit I needed to take it easy. By that evening, the pain was starting to come back. Not as bad as before, but definitely there.

I sat on my porch, a specialized Reparel compression sleeve on my elbow, laughing at myself. How many times had

I counseled patients through this exact scenario? How many times had I said, "Listen to your body, not your ego?"

Now, when patients hit setbacks during their recovery, I don't just *say* I understand — I *do* understand. I can empathetically say, "I've been there. I've felt your frustration, your fear that you've undone all your progress." But I also know what happens next if they trust the process and listen to their V-Motion Fit certified expert.

## Back to Full Strength

I backed off, followed my own V-Motion Fit team's protocols, and let my body heal at its own pace. By week twelve, I was at 95 percent recovery.

The real test came at Christmas. Lyla had grown and was now more than twenty pounds of squirming, excited, toddler energy. As I lifted her up to see the Christmas tree, I realized that I had no pain in my arm. Not even a twinge.

For the first time in twelve years, I was truly pain-free.

"There's never a *perfect* time," my wife had said. "Just do it."

She was right. While I'd been waiting for the perfect moment, I'd been missing life's perfect moments. Now I can hold my granddaughter, operate without compromise, and yes, I'm still making amazing pizzas. Just with better form.

# THE STORIES WE TELL OURSELVES

Here's what I've learned from treating thousands of patients and from being one myself: The things we tell ourselves about why we can't heal? Most of them just aren't true. Let me share five of the most common misbeliefs I hear patients say every day in my practice, and what the science actually tells us about your potential for healing.

> *The things we tell ourselves about why we can't heal? Most of them just aren't true.*

## Misbelief #1: "I'm too old."

Margaret was 89 when she told me she was too old to bother with repairing her joints. She'd been living with hip pain for three years, convinced that age meant accepting limitations. "Doctor," she said, "I'm too old for this to work."

Research shows that stem cell activity does decline with age, but it doesn't disappear. In fact, patients in their 80s and 90s still have significant regenerative capacity.[12] Margaret's outcome proved what data already told us was possible. After working with Victory In Motion, she returned to her morning walks and weekly grocery shopping. Age is just a number on your medical chart. Your cells don't check your birth certificate before repairing the joints in your body that need to be healed.

*Age is just a number on your medical chart. Your cells don't check your birth certificate before repairing the joints in your body that need to be healed.*

## Misbelief #2: "My damage is too far gone."

Remember Jean from the last chapter? Bone-on-bone arthritis, 82 years old, and told she *needed* surgery. Her repaired knee now works better and, according to her, "feels more normal" than her replaced one.

Even suffering from severe cartilage loss doesn't mean your case is hopeless. Through The Victory Method Programs, we're often treating your underlying bone issues that created the cartilage problem in the first place. This is the key to long-term healing.

## Misbelief #3: "I've already tried everything."

"Physical therapy, cortisone shots, pain pills, gel injections — nothing worked," Emilio said, listing off his treatments.

But when I asked about regenerative medicine, genetic-based nutrition, or comprehensive movement analysis, he'd never heard of them.

Ask yourself: Have you really tried everything?

The medical system offers a very limited menu of one-size-fits-all, insurance-based physical therapy, pain pills that damage your stomach and make you dizzy, messy ointments that stain your clothes, cortisone shots that damage cartilage, and gel shots that don't treat underlying bone problems.

After all those generic treatments fail to remove your pain, improve your range of motion, and restore your quality of life, you're told your options are either total joint replacement or to just "suck it up" and live with the pain. That's like being told by a food critic that you've tried every restaurant in town when you've really only been to three fast food chains.

## Misbelief #4: "Surgery is my only real option."

Says who? The same system that profits from surgery?

Remember Bill? He was told the same thing about his shoulder after a previous failed surgery. When Bill began working through The Victory Method, we treated his shoulder alongside his knees — no surgery required. The orthopedic industry performs between 800,000 and 1 million knee replacements annually, but studies show 25–30 percent may be unnecessary.[13] Because of this, it's always worth getting a second, or even a third, opinion.

## Misbelief #5: "This isn't the right time."

When is the right time to address constant, debilitating pain? When you can't walk at all? When you've missed your grandchild's first steps? When you're always the slow one lagging behind friends and family? When you can't go on that trip of a lifetime? When you can't enjoy the retirement funds you worked so hard to save? When you've given up everything you love?

I was a good example of falling into this misbelief myself. Now I can assure you both personally and professionally that there's never a perfect time to prioritize your health. There's only now.

## BREAKING THROUGH YOUR OWN BARRIERS

Lying in bed that first night after the procedure to repair the tendon in my elbow, doubting everything, tossing and turning, I learned that fear is normal. Doubt is human. The question isn't how to avoid these feelings; it's whether you'll let them stop you.

Your body wants to heal. It's designed to heal. The regenerative medicine process experienced by thousands of our patients follows predictable biological pathways. Growth factors activate within minutes to hours after the procedure. Stem cells, and other cells that help the stem cells, begin their work within hours to days. New tissue formation peaks around weeks four to eight.[14] Even with all of these cellular processes happening behind the scenes to repair your joint, your body needs the right support, the right environment, and most importantly, your belief that healing is possible.

Every patient whose story I've shared faced the same doubts you're facing. Bill was convinced nothing could help after his botched shoulder surgery. Jean swore she'd never go through another procedure. Even I, knowing everything I know, almost let fear keep me from healing.

But we all had one thing in common: we decided to trust the process more than we trusted our fear.

## THE REAL QUESTION

So, let me ask you what my wife essentially asked me: How long are you willing to live with limitations?

Not because you have to, but because you're afraid to believe things could be different?

How many more mornings will you choose to wake up in pain, telling yourself, "Maybe tomorrow"?

How many more activities will you give up, convincing yourself you're "too old" for them anyway? (Something we addressed in Misbelief #1.)

How many more moments will you miss because you're waiting for the "right time"?

Your body is remarkably resilient. Your capacity to heal is greater than you've been told — at *any* age. The only thing truly holding you back might be the story you're telling yourself about what's possible.

I'm not saying it will always be easy. I'm saying it's 100 percent *possible* (Not 100 percent guaranteed; only death and taxes fit that category.). And sometimes, that's all we need to know to take the first step.

If I can overcome my own limiting beliefs and walk this path, then you can too.

In the next chapter, I want to show you exactly what that path looks like. Not the theory, but the actual journey from where you are now to where you want to be. Because once you see the map, the only question left is whether you're ready to take the first step. Do you want to hear more about that pathway? Good, let's do it.

# CHAPTER 5

# YOUR VICTORY JOURNEY

Randi stood on the volcanic rocks of the Galápagos, her granddaughters' small hands warm in hers. Prickly pear cacti lined the beach like sentries. The colors surrounding them were otherworldly: rust-red lava flows, emerald-green highlands, and pale-gold grasses.

"Grandma, look at those birds on the beach!" Emma shouted, pointing excitedly. "They walk so funny, and they have blue feet!"

Randi smiled, her heart full. "Those are blue-footed boobies."

Claire started giggling at their name. Emma joined in, and soon, both girls were laughing uncontrollably, their joy echoing across the pristine beach.

This was paradise. Randi was living her dream of walking hand-in-hand with her granddaughters on the family trip they'd planned for years. The girls suddenly let go and scampered off, chasing the awkward birds along the shore.

Randi stepped off the rock to follow them, landing squarely on her left foot. A searing pain shot through her left knee like someone had just plunged a knife into it. She cried out and fell forward, face-first into the volcanic sand.

And then she woke from her dream.

Drenched in cold sweat, Randi gasped for air. Her husband, Steve, bolted upright beside her.

"Randi, are you okay?" he asked, half-asleep but fully alarmed. "It's your knee again, isn't it?"

Randi nodded, tears forming. "The Galápagos... I'm just not up to it. We'll have to cancel unless a miracle happens."

She sat silently, then looked at him with sudden determination. "I heard that Dr. Pietropaoli is using stem cell treatments to repair joints. Maybe that can be our miracle. I'm calling his office first thing in the morning."

That call changed everything for Randi.

## THE PATH FROM PAIN TO PARADISE

Here's what I've learned after helping thousands of patients: healing follows the same pathway, every time. I call this pathway The Victory Journey. Whether you're like Randi, fighting to reclaim your dreams of adventure, or you simply want to climb stairs without pain, your journey to healing will take you through five predictable stages.

The Victory Journey is your personal roadmap that will take you from where you are now to where you want to be — mobile, active, and living the life you deserve.

*The Victory Journey is your personal roadmap that will take you from where you are now to where you want to be — mobile, active, and living the life you deserve.*

Your body wants to heal. It's biologically programmed to repair itself. But it needs the right sequence, the right support, and the right environment. That's exactly what these five stages provide.

Let me show you how Randi, and hundreds of patients like her, transformed their lives by following this path.

# YOUR VICTORY JOURNEY™
## 5 Stages to Knee Repair, NOT Knee Replacement®

## LOCK IN RESULTS
### Make It Last
Maintain progress with sustainable habits, so your transformation lasts for years to come.

**5**

**4**

## REBUILD STRENGTH
### Support Your Healing
Restore movement, rebuild muscle, and retrain patterns so your healing becomes functional.

## ACTIVATE HEALING
### Give Your Body the Tools It Needs
Harness your own cells and healing factors to jump-start repair in bone, cartilage, and soft tissues.

**3**

**2**

## RESET & RECHARGE
### Prepare Your Body to Heal
Reduce inflammation and create the environment your body needs to respond to treatment.

**1**

## CLARITY DAY™
### Get Real Answers
Discover the true root causes of your pain through advanced imaging and a Comprehensive Diagnostic Evaluation™.

**START**

# STAGE 1: CLARITY DAY

Most treatments fail because they address symptoms, not root causes. Without knowing the true root causes of your pain, we're all just shooting in the dark.

When Randi called my office the morning after her nightmare, her desperation was palpable. "My left knee is literally killing me," she told Jamie, our patient care coordinator. "I want the stem cells that my friend Louise told me about. She'd also been told she had to have a knee replaced, and your team prevented her from needing that painful surgery."

"I have a family trip of a lifetime coming up in seven months to the Galápagos Islands," Randi explained. "My husband, Steve, and I have been saving and planning this trip for years. We've already spent thousands of dollars on it, and now I'm terrified I won't be able to go."

That's when she learned about the Clarity Day — our way of getting to the root of what's really happening in a patient's body to understand what's causing their pain. After Jamie finished telling Randi about the Clarity Day, she immediately enrolled in our program.

## The Science Behind Stage 1

Advanced imaging reveals problems and issues in joints that standard x-rays and many standard MRIs cannot. A specialized MRI can detect bone marrow lesions and microfractures that are completely invisible to routine exams. These "soft spots" in the bone not only cause most of the pain from arthritis, but they also indicate a nine times higher risk of needing joint replacement.[15]

Randi's Clarity Day experience was transformational. Her Comprehensive Diagnostic Evaluation revealed inflammation patterns, movement dysfunctions, and underlying bone issues that explained why standard treatments had failed her. For the first time in months, she had hope based on facts, not guesswork.

### What This Means for You

Instead of blindly moving forward with a treatment plan just because it's what everybody else thinks is the only way forward, a Clarity Day allows you to know *exactly* what is going on with your body, the root causes of your symptoms, and the proven steps that have transformed others with those same conditions.

## STAGE 2: RESET AND RECHARGE

Before any garden can flourish, you must prepare the soil. Your body is no different. It can't heal in an inflammatory environment. Stage 2 removes the physiological obstacles that impede healing and optimizes your cellular function.

## VICTORY METHOD™ PROGRAM
### Growth Progress to Pain Relief

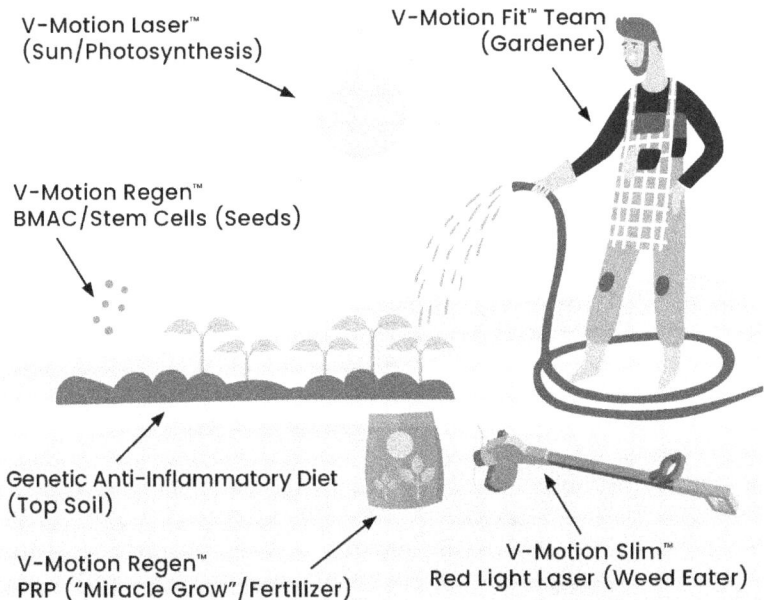

V-Motion Laser™
(Sun/Photosynthesis)

V-Motion Fit™ Team
(Gardener)

V-Motion Regen™
BMAC/Stem Cells (Seeds)

Genetic Anti-Inflammatory Diet
(Top Soil)

V-Motion Regen™
PRP ("Miracle Grow"/Fertilizer)

V-Motion Slim™
Red Light Laser (Weed Eater)

For Randi, her resetting process began with a comprehensive DNA analysis and comprehensive lab work that revealed surprising truths about her metabolism. "I thought I was eating healthy," she admitted when she got her results. "Turns out, half of what I considered 'good foods' like seed oils, many types of yogurts that have a lot of hidden added sugar, and even whole wheat bread, were actually increasing my inflammation."

## The Science Behind Stage 2

Chronic inflammation blocks stem cell activity and disrupts the healing cascade. Numerous studies have shown that reducing systemic inflammation can improve stem cell activity and regenerative medicine therapies.[16]

Over the next three weeks, Randi eliminated specific inflammatory foods identified by her genetic profile and comprehensive blood work. She began taking specific dietary supplements to promote healthy digestion, detox, weight loss, vitality, and energy. She also started red light laser therapy sessions, which she later described to her husband, Steve, in this way:

"It's like science fiction," she told him. "You just lie there while this light works on opening your fat cells, allowing the inflammatory fat to drain away and be eliminated by your body naturally. There are no needles, no pain, and nothing invasive, but I feel as though I can actually feel the inflammation going away."

"The weirdest part?" she added, "I started sleeping through the night. I hadn't realized how much the inflammation was affecting my entire system."

## What This Means for You

Your knee doesn't exist in isolation. Systemic inflammation creates an environment where healing can't occur. The Reset and Recharge stage of The Victory Journey prepares your body to actually respond to treatment.

Reducing the inflammation in your body also positively influences your cardiovascular system, brain and nervous system, immune system, metabolic system, gut health, skin, and lung health. It also reduces the risk of cancer and improves overall longevity and quality of life. Amazing! Don't you agree?

## STAGE 3: ACTIVATE HEALING

Your body has remarkable healing capacity, but sometimes it requires biological reinforcement. The third stage of The Victory Journey provides concentrated healing factors and cells exactly where they're needed. Cells do the work and are analogous to the seeds in a garden. PRP is analogous to "Miracle-Gro" fertilizer. We use the red light laser in Stage 2 to decrease fat and inflammation. Inflammation is kind of like weeds in a garden. Weeds choke out the good plants, and inflammation chokes out our cells from healing. We use a deep tissue healing laser, which is a separate type of laser compared to the red light fat loss laser from Stage 2. Healing laser therapy is analogous to sunlight, which helps plants grow. Photosynthesis for plants in the garden is analogous to photobiomodulation in the human body.

With her inflammation under control, Randi's body was finally ready to heal. This is where regenerative medicine works its magic.

Randi's biggest fear was the bone marrow harvest. "Does it hurt?" she asked nervously, just like almost every other patient we work with.

"There's definitely some discomfort," our team member, Allison, explained, "but we use long-acting local anesthetic. Even Dr. P had this procedure done, and he said it felt more weird than painful."

## The Science Behind Stage 3

Bone marrow concentrate contains multiple cell types, including stem cells, which work synergistically to jump-start the healing process in cartilage, bone, muscles, tendons, and other soft tissues, while simultaneously reducing inflammation and promoting repair and growth.

When the day of her procedure arrived, Randi was nervous but excited. "I thought this was going to be much harder," she said once we'd finished. "I felt a little pop, like you told me I would, but it was only slightly uncomfortable when you pulled out the bone marrow cells. It was more weird than painful, just like you said."

Less than an hour later, Randi's husband arrived to pick her up, and the only visible signs of her procedure were gauze and an ACE bandage wrapped around her knee as she walked out the door.

"I thought they were going to have to bring you out in a wheelchair," Steve said, amazed.

"Nope," Randi smiled. "Walk in and walk out!"

## What This Means for You

Your body wants to heal; it just needs the right tools and the right place. Regenerative medicine treatments like laser therapy, PRP, and bone marrow cells are definitely not experimental; they simply use your body's own repair mechanisms — with help from us — where they're needed most.

# STAGE 4: REBUILD STRENGTH

Regenerative therapy provides the biological foundation for healing, but lasting recovery requires rebuilding the supporting structures around your joint. Unfortunately, this is where many regenerative programs fail, because they stop after the injection. But healing cells, growth factors, and lasers are only part of the equation.

Stage 4 of The Victory Journey is where patients like Jerry, a golf professional, and many other golf professionals and everyday golfers we treat, demonstrate what's possible. At 72, Jerry came to me facing a crisis that threatened everything he'd built his life around.

"Golf isn't just my career," he told me, his voice breaking slightly. "It's who I am. If I can't rotate my hips properly, I can't teach." He paused, staring at his hands. "And if I can't teach, who am I?"

Jerry had degeneration in both knees that was affecting his hip and back rotation and vice versa — a vicious cycle that was severely impacting his quality of life. Standing for golf lessons was agony. Demonstrating swings was impossible. He'd already canceled two teaching clinics, something he'd never done in four decades.

"I'm scared," he admitted. "I see these young instructors coming up, all technology and TrackMan data. The only thing I have that they don't is experience. But if I can't perform, what good is experience?"

## The Science Behind Stage 4

Muscle atrophy begins quickly when activity drops, and it's detectable within about 48 hours of immobilization.[17] The good news is that targeted strengthening and movement retraining can restore function even when there's structural wear. In knee osteoarthritis, programs that retrain gait or neuromuscular control decrease the mechanical loading forces on the joint during walking, which helps reduce pain and can make a joint feel younger.

Both Randi and Jerry entered our V-Motion Fit total-body fitness program after the first three stages of their regenerative treatments, but their paths differed when it came to rebuilding strength based on their unique needs and goals.

Randi's V-Motion Fit program focused on rebuilding the supporting muscles around her knee and the rest of her body. Also, correcting movement patterns that contributed to her degeneration and prepared her for the uneven terrain she'd encounter in her upcoming Galápagos dream vacation.

Jerry's journey was about precision and performance. Every exercise was designed to restore the specific movement patterns golf demanded while protecting his healing joints.

"I hit a wall around week six," Randi admitted. "The progress slowed, and I started wondering if I'd made a mistake not getting the surgery."

Jerry faced his own crisis of faith. "My knees felt better, but my swing still wasn't right. I had a tournament coming up that I'd been teaching at for fifteen years. The thought of canceling was killing me."

This is normal. Healing is not linear. The biological healing process follows predictable phases, but functional recovery requires patience and persistence.

# YOUR RECOVERY JOURNEY

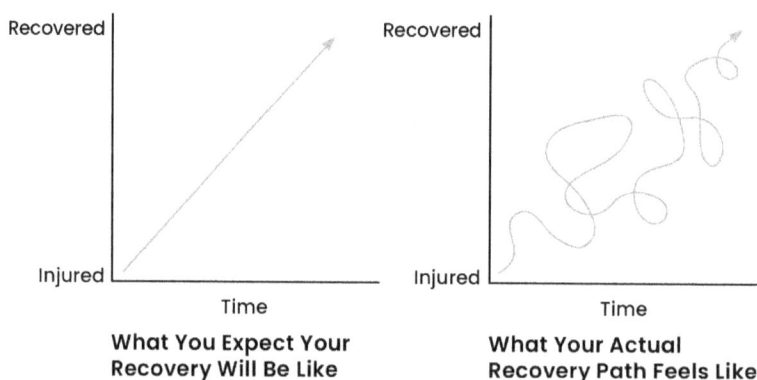

**What You Expect Your Recovery Will Be Like**

**What Your Actual Recovery Path Feels Like**

Both patients pushed through. Randi's first breakthrough came during week eight when she climbed the stairs at her office without thinking about it. "When I got to the top and realized I hadn't held the rail, I actually teared up."

Jerry's moment arrived on the driving range during week ten. "I'd been protecting my back, hip, and knees for so long, I'd forgotten how to trust my body. Then one morning, everything clicked. The rotation, the power, the follow-through — it all came back."

But his real transformation went deeper. "I lost 47 pounds and discovered muscles I never knew I had. The strength training and movement correction weren't just about my knees; it changed my entire body. I feel 20 years younger!" he told me later.

"My girlfriend Karen was so impressed, she also underwent one of your Victory Method programs due to pain from arthritis in her right knee. She was able to reach her goals of walking three miles a day with her friends, golfing without pain, playing pickleball, hiking and maintaining her active lifestyle. Most importantly, we avoided knee replacements. If we can do it, anyone can do it."

And Randi ultimately did so well that her husband, Steve, also underwent a Knee Repair, NOT Knee Replacement program for both of his knees and was able to get back to golf and hiking.

### What This Means for You

Regenerative medicine therapy gives your body the tools to heal. V-Motion Fit gives you the strength to use that healing. Without both, you're only getting half the solution.

## STAGE 5: LOCK IN RESULTS

Success isn't just about reaching your goal; it's about maintaining it. The fifth stage of The Victory Journey ensures your physical improvement and your changed habits become your new normal.

Jerry chose our Supported Maintenance plan, which included monthly check-ins, quarterly laser "tune-ups," and ongoing nutrition and V-Motion Fit guidance. "I invested too much in getting better to let it slip away," he reasoned.

Randi opted for our Independent Maintenance plan and was equipped with a home fitness and mobility program and the knowledge she needed to manage her own care. "I know my body now in a way I never did before," she said.

## The Science Behind Stage 5

Improvements from bone marrow aspirate cells and PRP can persist for years in many patients.[18] But the biggest predictor of staying better after treatment is turning movement and anti-inflammatory nutrition into habits. Randomized trials and long-term studies show that patients who sustain exercise and effective weight management over 12–24 months maintain greater pain relief and function than those who stop.[19]

Both approaches work. The key is choosing what fits your lifestyle and goals.

## What This Means for You

Whether your maintenance plan is supported or independent, your commitment to maintaining your transformation and continually moving forward in your Victory Method Program will ensure your success for years to come.

# TWO VICTORIES, ONE PATHWAY

Randi's true breakthrough moment came during a trip to a waterpark with her grandkids. As they packed up after a full day of walking and playing, her son turned to her and said, "Mom, do you realize you walked around all day today and didn't complain about your knee once?"

She paused, looked at him, and smiled. "That was my aha moment," she said. "That's when I knew it had worked."

Jerry's victory was different but equally powerful. Six months after starting his journey, he not only returned to teaching golf full-time, but also won a regional senior championship. "The tournament was the proof," he said. "It was proof not just that I could play again, but that I could compete. I wasn't just surviving, I was thriving."

Ten months after Randi woke from her nightmare in a cold sweat, she stood on the volcanic shores of the Galápagos Islands. Not in a dream, in reality. She laughed as Emma and Claire giggled about blue-footed boobies and ran after the awkward birds. She stepped off the rock to follow them.

This time, there was no pain. Just paradise — and a *huge* smile!

Meanwhile, Jerry returned to the life he'd built around golf with new wisdom. "I tell all my fellow pros not to wait until surgery is their only option," he says. "The Victory Method Journey doesn't just fix the problem; it makes you better than you were before."

## WHERE THEY ARE TODAY

Today, Randi moves freely between her homes in New York and Florida. She runs up and down stairs to her boat without a second thought. "The only thing holding me back now," she laughs, "is the Florida heat and my hormones — but that's a different chapter."

Jerry continues teaching golf and competing at the highest level. He's become an advocate for The Victory Method among his professional golf colleagues and especially his students. "I see too many pros and my students pushing through pain, thinking they just need to 'tough it out,'" he says. "I tell them that there *is* a better way. Don't wait until you're facing surgery."

Both patients represent something important: The Victory Journey doesn't just help fix what's broken; it often makes you function better than you did before your pain started.

"I understand my body now," Randi reflects. "I know what it needs to thrive, not just survive."

Jerry agrees: "My swing is more efficient now. My teaching is better because I understand movement and recovery in a way I never did before."

## YOUR JOURNEY STARTS WITH A SINGLE STEP

Every patient's Victory Journey is unique, but the pathway is proven. Whether you're like Randi, fighting to reclaim dreams of adventure and family experiences, or like Jerry, determined to maintain professional performance, the five stages remain the same:

1. **Get clarity** about what's really happening in your body.
2. **Reset** your internal environment to allow healing.
3. **Activate** your body's regenerative potential.
4. **Rebuild** your strength and function.
5. **Lock in** your results for lasting success.

The journey typically takes 12 to 16 weeks, though some patients see dramatic improvement sooner, while others need more time. What matters isn't the exact timeline; it's the transformation that fits your specific goals and lifestyle.

Randi's closing words stay with me: "I spent so long accepting limitations, believing that aging meant giving up the things I loved. You showed me another way. The dream I thought was dying was just waiting for me to be brave enough to pursue it."

Jerry put it differently but with equal conviction: "I almost let fear make the decision for me. I almost chose surgery because it seemed like the 'safe' option. But this gave me something surgery never could: a body that's actually stronger and more resilient than before."

Your dreams are waiting too. Randi and Jerry proved The Victory Journey works for people from all walks of life with

different goals, different challenges, and different defini-
tions of success. Whether you're dreaming of walking volcanic beaches with your grandchildren or sinking the perfect
putt, whether you're 45 or 85, whether your goals are athletic
performance or simply walking without pain, the pathway
is the same.

Every Victory Journey begins with clarity. Because until
you truly understand what's happening in your body — and
what needs to be corrected — it's easy to stay stuck in the
same old cycle of temporary fixes and mounting limitations.
That's why Clarity Day matters so much. It's not just the first
step. It's the step that makes every other step possible.

In the next chapter, I'll show you exactly what happens on
a Clarity Day and why it's the most important thing you can
do to finally start moving forward.

# CHAPTER 6

# WE START
# WITH CLARITY

After 27 years of practicing medicine, I've learned something important: most people don't need more treatment options; they just need to understand exactly what's wrong. That's where everything starts.

Too many patients come to me after months — sometimes years — of guessing. They've tried pills, shots, and standard physical therapy based on incomplete information. They've been told they need surgery without anyone taking the time to show them what's actually happening inside their joint or damaged body part.

The problem with guessing is that when you don't know precisely what's going on and *why*, you end up treating symptoms instead of coming up with solutions. But when we know the exact root causes of your condition, we can design an individualized treatment plan, which we cannot do with patients who do not undergo a Comprehensive Diagnostic Evaluation during a Clarity Day.

> *The problem with guessing is that when you don't know precisely what's going on and why, you end up treating symptoms instead of coming up with solutions.*

That's one of the primary reasons I developed The Victory Journey, and why your first step on that journey is to get clarity about the root causes of your condition. And you want these answers fast. Who wants to wait weeks, months, years — or worse, *forever* — to figure out exactly what's wrong with them?

In the previous chapter, I showed you the five stages of The Victory Journey. Now let's zoom in on Stage 1: Clarity Day, the essential first step of the process, so you can see how it greatly increases your chances for success.

I designed Clarity Day to give you answers fast without the months of delays, referrals, and insurance battles — something we call the "Cycle of Insanity" that frustrate so many patients.

The day unfolds step by step, each building on the last, so by the end, you and I have a complete picture of what's happening in your body and how to fix it.

Let me tell you about Katie and how this one day changed the trajectory of her entire recovery. Here's how Katie's Clarity Day unfolded, and how yours will too.

## KATIE'S LEAP OF FAITH

At 59, Katie was the kind of person who made fitness look effortless. She hiked every weekend, attended CrossFit religiously, and could outlast most people half her age on a long walk. During COVID-19, she'd stayed active, but over time, her workouts became sporadic. Her muscles stiffened. Her mobility declined.

Looking back, Katie realized the warning signs had been there for months. The subtle hip discomfort after her weekend hikes. The tightness that settled in after long hours at her desk. She had to stretch a little longer each morning just to feel normal.

"I thought I was just getting older," she told me. "Or that maybe I needed to get in better shape."

She felt off but didn't know how off she really was until one joyful moment turned into one of her most painful.

Katie had just flown into Newark Airport from Charlotte, North Carolina, where she'd attended a business trip, when a dear friend she hadn't seen in years spotted her outside baggage claim. Overcome with excitement, her friend swept her up in one of those enthusiastic bear hugs that lift you completely off your feet. Overcome with joy, her friend shook her back and forth.

And just like that, something tore deep inside her right hip.

The pain was immediate and blinding. She felt something rip — not a twinge or a pull, but a sharp, unmistakable tear that took her breath away.

She pushed through dinner that night, hiding her agony behind smiles and conversation. But when she was alone in her hotel room, she knew something was very wrong. Every step sent lightning through her pelvis. Sitting was excruciating. Standing was worse.

The flight home the next morning was torture. She limped through the airport, struggling with her luggage, too proud to ask for help. "I didn't want to be one of *those people* who needed assistance," she said. "But I was hoping someone would notice how much pain I was in."

Whether your own pain has been gradually growing, or, like Katie, a specific trauma has made it unbearable, and you've tried to get help from the traditional medical system, you will probably recognize what happened next.

Her first visit was to urgent care, where she was simply dismissed. "You're just sore," the PA told her. "Take some ibuprofen."

Friends offered well-meaning advice and said, "You probably just tweaked something. It'll heal on its own." Even people she trusted seemed to minimize what she knew was serious damage.

"I started to wonder if I was being dramatic," she told me. "But I knew something wasn't right."

She had become "that person" who limped through crowds, slowing everyone down and needing help instead of being independent. What terrified her even more was her future: More pain, more delays, and maybe even a hip replacement.

Through endless nights of pain and frustration, Katie finally made a bold decision: "I don't care what it costs. I'm contacting Dr. P."

## WHAT HAPPENS ON YOUR CLARITY DAY

Katie had connections in the regenerative medicine world and had been following my work online for more than a year. The morning after her declaration, she booked a telecommunication consult.

Speaking with Katie, it became clear she was in significant pain and that we would be able to help. As soon as the interview was complete, she booked a flight to Syracuse for her Clarity Day. The next morning, she arrived at our office early, filled with both excitement and apprehension about the unknown.

Here's exactly what Katie experienced, and what you can expect during your comprehensive evaluation:

### 9:00 a.m. to 10:00 a.m.: Provider Consultation

We started Katie's Clarity Day with a thorough regenerative medicine consultation. This isn't a typical, seven-minute appointment; it's a comprehensive session with me or one of our expert regenerative medicine medical providers. You may even eventually visit a clinic that we have trained and certified on our Victory Method.

When I sat down across from Katie, her eyes were red from crying, and I could see her weariness from travel and lack of sleep. But once we made eye contact, her demeanor gradually shifted to one of hopefulness that grew as I asked her questions that mapped out her injury history, her goals, and exactly what had happened at that airport.

Most providers never learn what you actually want to achieve. They treat the diagnosis, not your dreams. With The Victory Method, we help you define clear goals for your treatment so you can live the life you want to live.

Several times during her history and comprehensive musculoskeletal physical exam, Katie commented, "The urgent care staff didn't do a total-body physical exam like you and your team did here; they just poked at my hip a little."

"Unfortunately, we hear that all the time," I told her. "But it's not necessarily those other providers' fault. That type of care is the result of a system that is reactive and favors quantity over quality."

> *Most providers never learn what you actually want to achieve. They treat the diagnosis, not your dreams. With The Victory Method, we help you define clear goals for your treatment so you can live the life you want to live.*

## 10:00 a.m. to 10:30 a.m.: Digital Imaging and Live Ultrasound

Next came immediate digital x-rays, performed quickly and efficiently by Stephanie, one of our radiology techs, followed by live ultrasound imaging performed by me.

Real-time ultrasound reveals soft tissue damage invisible on x-rays. We can see inflammation patterns, arthritic changes, meniscus cartilage damage, muscle, tendon, or ligament tears, and joint fluid changes that will explain your symptoms without having to wait for the images to be printed and delivered for assessment.

"Fortunately," I told Katie, "your x-rays don't show any fractures or arthritis, which is great. But let's take a better look at your muscles. The gel is going to be a little cold, but there shouldn't be any pain as I perform the ultrasound."

As I gently placed the ultrasound transducer over her black and blue upper thigh, Katie could actually see what was happening inside her hip for the first time since her injury occurred. "Look," I said, "that black area is blood from your torn muscle. It's what we call a hematoma."

"So, I'm *not* crazy," she whispered, pointing at the monitor. "It's really torn. But if there's no arthritis, I won't have to have my hip replaced, right?"

"That's right," I said.

No more guessing.

## 10:30 a.m. to Noon: Bathroom break and MRI Confirmation

After a short break, Addison, a radiology tech, came into the exam room and led Katie to the Open MRI suite. Katie said, "Now? Today? It usually takes three weeks just to get the insurance authorization back home in Charlotte."

Addison told her that the average wait time for an MRI can be weeks to months. "The beauty of a Clarity Day is that we're able to perform the MRI, have it read by a board-certified radiologist, and Dr. P. or Jordan, our physician assistant, can go over it with you all in the same day!"

Delayed diagnosis means delayed healing.

Unlike an x-ray, MRIs show the soft tissues, like cartilage, muscles, tendons, and ligaments, as well as stress/microfractures, which are soft spots in the supporting bone under the cartilage that are the main cause of pain from arthritis.

I told Katie, "If the bone under the cartilage, the subchondral bone, gets soft, then there is no support for the overlying cartilage, and the cartilage starts to break down. That cartilage breaking down on the end of the bone is the arthritis. This process is exactly like how a pothole in the road develops. The underlayer of the road washes away, leaving less support for the overlying asphalt pavement, which leads to the pavement breaking down and a pothole forming."

For Katie, the images confirmed what we suspected. She had no bone or cartilage damage, but there was a significant muscle tear that would require regenerative medicine treatment to give it the best chance to heal properly without surgery.

## 12:00 p.m. to 1:00 p.m.: Lunch

Victory In Motion is located in Skaneateles, New York, which is a beautiful vacation destination in the Finger Lakes. We encourage our patients to explore the area and get a bite to eat at one of the many wonderful dining establishments. We have many great recommendations, and lunch is on us!

## 1:00 p.m. to 2:00 p.m.: V-Motion Fit Functional Total-Body Fitness Assessment

It wouldn't be surprising if we found that your joint conditions have led to musculoskeletal issues, such as poor movement patterns, stability problems, or muscle weaknesses. As we grow older, these musculoskeletal issues place more stress on joints and contribute to greater pain or injury.

Because of this, after her lunch break, our total-body fitness, strength and conditioning specialists put Katie through a comprehensive movement evaluation, including a Functional Movement Screen, range of motion test, and a head-to-toe strength, stability, and mechanical assessment.

The assessment revealed moderate to severe weaknesses of her back and lower legs that had made her susceptible to her hip injury. Now Katie began to understand why this had happened.

## 2:00 p.m. to 3:00 p.m.: Team Consultation and Treatment Planning

By late afternoon, our physician assistant, Jordan; our V-Motion Fit specialist, Lucci; our scribe, Allison; and I sat down with Katie to review her Clarity Day Comprehensive Diagnostic Evaluation results.

No pressure. No rush. Just information delivered in plain language so she could make a confident decision.

We revisited her goals, including her dreams, her business commitments, and her upcoming family events, and explored what "feeling better" would truly mean for her life. We explained that we never hand out cookie-cutter, inject-and-go, a la carte treatments like so many regenerative medicine clinics do.

Like all of our programs, every option we offered to Katie was built on these three pillars:

1. **The patient's medical findings** from the Comprehensive Diagnostic Evaluation, including their medical history, comprehensive physical exam, x-ray and ultrasound findings, AI Open MRI results, total-body fitness evaluation, and list of goals and dreams.
2. **The patient's ability to commit time** to their recovery and how much time.
3. **The patient's financial situation** and the level of investment in the program fit their comfort level.

We laid out three comprehensive, whole-person programs that we call our "good, better, best" options. There is also a **destination overseas Caribbean clinic option.** We emphasized that all of these were personally designed to help her heal and return to the activities she loved, and that the differences came down to the level of intensity, biological support, total-body resources, and financial investment in each tier.

Katie chose to be treated in the US. Her good, better, best options looked like this:

- **Good**: *Provides a strong starting point for healing.*
  - » For Katie, this option would start with a PRP injection, followed by 12 combined V-Motion Fit and healing V- Motion laser sessions.

- **Better**: *Includes more biological support, extended total-body rehab, and long-term follow-up.*
  - » Katie was told this would include an injection of bone marrow aspirate cells and PRP, followed by 24 V-Motion Fit and healing laser therapy sessions. After this, she'd get a one-year follow-up

membership with ongoing progress reviews and other member perks.

- **Best**: *Maximum intensity, personalization, and access to advanced care.*
  - » Katie's "best" option included everything from the first two tiers, plus V-Motion Slim, which includes a DNA-based, anti-inflammatory nutrition program with three months of one-on-one guidance from a registered dietitian, along with red light laser treatment appointments for anti-inflammatory fat and weight loss.

We stressed that these programs were not generic — they were personalized for her unique medical findings, lifestyle demands, and personal aspirations.

As we talked, Katie asked thoughtful questions about recovery time, rehabilitation, financing (which is an option), and ongoing care. One of her concerns was that because she traveled a lot, she would not be able to attend 24 in-person V-Motion Fit and deep tissue healing laser treatments after her injections.

I firmly believe that something good always comes out of something bad. COVID-19 was a good example of that. Many bad things happened during that time, but one good thing to come out of the COVID-19 pandemic was widespread use and acceptance of telemedicine. Because we don't offer cookie-cutter care, we further customized Katie's program to make the majority of her V-Motion Fit visits telemedicine, since we had become experts at telemedicine in the early 2020s.

To address Katie's travel concerns, we substituted a hand-held healing laser for the in-person laser treatments, and after weighing her options, Katie chose the customized, modified "Better-plus" program that would give her body the biological tools it needed to heal her tear properly — a combination of targeted injections, about 12 weeks of 24 telemedicine V-Motion Fit appointments, prescribed daily handheld laser treatments, and a personalized, genetic-based, anti-inflammatory nutrition plan.

As it was for Katie, by choosing the specific program that *you* believe is best for your situation and goals, you are making a full commitment to your health, your life, and your future.

## 3:30 p.m. to 4:30 p.m. Treatment and Recovery

After Katie chose her specific program, we performed the bone marrow aspirate concentrate and PRP procedure that very afternoon. Using ultrasound guidance, and without making any incisions, we administered two small injections and applied a couple of Band-Aids afterward. It's not always possible for this procedure to be performed on the same day as the patient's Clarity Day, but we do our best to provide as much care as possible in a single-day experience.

Katie stayed in town for two days of additional healing with deep tissue laser treatments and in-person V-Motion Fit training. Can you see how we use the same general principles and pillars of The Victory Method, but customize them to your specific personal needs?

She then continued her recovery program from her home a thousand miles away via telemedicine appointments with the V-Motion Fit team twice a week; daily, self-administered handheld healing laser treatments; and monthly follow-ups with me.

Katie's journey wasn't perfectly smooth, because real healing rarely is. It was a journey of ups and downs, but fortunately, with The Victory Method, there are more ups than downs!

A few weeks into her recovery, she skipped some of her prescribed exercises and felt a sharp pain during a yoga class. Panic set in immediately.

"Did I re-tear it?" she asked during an emergency telemedicine call.

This is another point in her journey where the traditional medical system would have failed her. She would have waited days or weeks for an appointment, probably ended up in urgent care, and likely been told she needed to start over with a different specialist.

Instead, we adjusted her program that same day. I reassured her that setbacks are normal and explained that her injured tissues were indeed healing, but still weak and prone to reinjury. So, we advised her to continue her prescribed V-Motion Fit exercises as ordered.

The breakthrough came eight weeks later when Katie returned to our office. Her follow-up MRI revealed the tear had almost completely healed. When I pointed out the change in her before-and-after images, she started crying.

"I can see it," she said. "I'm not imagining this. It's actually working."

That emotional moment, seeing proof of her body's healing, allowed Katie to finally alleviate much of her worry and trust that she was healing, stop second-guessing the process, and commit fully to the remaining V-Motion Fit sessions.

By the 12-week mark, she returned to her yoga class with a confidence she'd never had before. "I'm not afraid of my body anymore," she told me. "My right hip is actually better than my left now. I didn't realize how tight that other side had become."

## FINDING CLARITY TOGETHER

Not every patient comes to us in a moment of crisis like Katie did. Sometimes people find us after years of chronic frustration with the traditional system. These people rarely come alone. As a matter of fact, we *require* you to bring a spouse, partner, loved one, parent, sibling, child, or close friend so you are not alone in this process and have support before, during, and after the program starts. It is always great to have an extra set of ears on your team, since we go over so much information during your full Clarity Day.

Tom and Linda had been married for 34 years when Tom reached his breaking point with his hip and knee pain.

According to his orthopedist, they were "bone-on-bone," and insisted he needed replacement surgery.

Tom had been through the familiar cycle: cortisone shots that provided temporary relief, physical therapy that felt like going through the motions, gel injections that didn't help, and pain medications that made him feel foggy or, according to him, "ripped my stomach apart."

"I was miserable," Tom told me later. "And I was making Linda miserable too because I was complaining all the time, but I wouldn't do anything about it."

Linda had been watching her husband struggle for months. "His pain was keeping us both up at night," she said. "I was worried about him, but I was also frustrated because nothing seemed to help."

When a friend told them about our Knee Repair, NOT Knee Replacement approach and the Clarity Day, they were skeptical but desperate enough to try.

"We just wanted to know what was really going on," Tom said. "We were nervous about what you'd find, but we were tired of guessing."

Linda insisted on coming with him to all his appointments, including his Clarity Day — a decision that proved to be exactly what was needed.

"The difference was immediate," Linda recalled. "We walked into the office expecting more of the same runaround, but instead we found a team that actually listened to both of us."

During Tom's Comprehensive Diagnostic Evaluation, both he and Linda learned things about his condition that no one had ever explained before. The digital imaging revealed not just the arthritis they knew about, but underlying bone issues that were contributing to his pain. Similarly, Tom's V-Motion Fit assessment showed functional problems that had never been identified.

"No one ever told us about the bone marrow microfractures and edema that were causing most of my arthritis pain," Tom said, referring to the soft spots we found in his knee bones. "Suddenly, everything made sense."

Linda was amazed by the thoroughness of the process. "In one day, you showed us more about what was wrong than we'd learned in months of other appointments," she said. "We knew his weight was a huge problem, but we didn't realize how it was not only increasing the stress on Tom's joints, but the inflammation throughout his body as well."

She added, "We knew inflammation was 'bad', but we didn't realize how chronic inflammation negatively affects every cell in our bodies. It was at the core of all of his *other* medical problems as well."

For the first time in years, they had clarity about what was actually wrong with Tom's entire body and what could be done about it. We presented them with realistic options, not just surgery or living with pain.

"You didn't pressure us at all," Linda recalled. "You just gave us information and let us decide."

After Tom's Clarity Day, they chose to proceed with one of our Victory Method programs. Six months later, Tom had dropped 113 pounds, and Linda was grateful to have her husband back. "Tom's primary care doctor was amazed at his total-body transformation and took him off all his blood pressure, cholesterol, and heart medications," she said.

"We just wish we'd done this sooner," they both told me at his follow-up appointment.

## WHY THIS COMPREHENSIVE APPROACH CAN TRANSFORM LIVES

Here's something most providers don't tell you: incomplete diagnosis is the leading cause of treatment failure. Research shows that when practitioners jump to treatment without understanding the full picture, success rates drop. In fact, delayed diagnosis can reduce or eliminate the possibility of non-surgical treatment for osteoarthritis.[20]

Think about it like this: If your car were making a noise, would you want a mechanic to start replacing parts without first figuring out what's causing the problem? Would you want to let the noise continue until it's too late to solve the problem at all? Unfortunately, that's exactly what happens in most medical offices. Well-meaning doctors, limited by the current medical system, treat your symptoms, maybe order an x-ray, hope for the best, and try something else when it fails.

On the other hand, The Victory Method is a comprehensive approach that identifies not just what hurts, but *why* it hurts.

The bone marrow microfractures Tom had? They are invisible on regular x-rays and can only be seen on specialized MRI sequences but are crucial for treatment planning. With Artificial Intelligence now built into our Victory AI Open MRI, what once took much longer can now be done in a fraction of the time, and with images so clear, even tiny microfractures become visible.

> *The Victory Method is a comprehensive approach that identifies not just what hurts, but why it hurts.*

The abnormal full-body movement patterns Katie developed? Standard physical therapy evaluations can miss those.

The systemic inflammation many patients carry? It never gets addressed in joint-focused treatments. Genetic testing and appropriate labs can identify this and many other issues as well.

When we understand the complete picture — joint health, bone quality, movement patterns, systemic factors — we can address the actual problem instead of just managing symptoms.

## CLARITY DAY SNAPSHOT

In case you need a quick reference, here's exactly what your Clarity Day includes:

## 60–90 Minute Provider Evaluation

You'll meet with an expert regenerative medicine medical provider for a comprehensive consultation. We'll review your complete past and current medical history, understand your goals, and perform a thorough physical examination. It's *not* the 10-minute appointment you're used to.

## Digital X-rays with Immediate Review

We'll perform new digital x-rays with specialized views you may not have had previously and review them with you immediately. You'll see exactly what's happening in your joint and understand what those images actually mean for your condition.

## Live Ultrasound Evaluation

Using real-time ultrasound, we'll examine your soft tissues, muscles, tendons, and joint health. You'll be able to see what's happening inside your body, live, as we explain it.

## Same-Day Open MRI

Same-day, custom MRI with special imaging sequences can identify stress/microfractures or soft spots in bones that can make you nine times more likely to need a joint replacement. Our non-claustrophobic, open MRI images are read that same day by a board-certified radiologist. AI will also be utilized to help assist in the interpretation of those MRI images in the very near future.

## V-Motion Fit Functional Assessment

Our total-body fitness strength and conditioning specialists will put you through a comprehensive evaluation of your strength, mobility, and functional and mechanical patterns.

This often reveals underlying issues that contribute to your pain but have never been identified.

## Complimentary Laser Therapy Session

You'll experience one of our advanced deep tissue healing laser treatments to immediately start reducing inflammation and supporting your body's natural healing process.

## 60–90-Minute Team Treatment Planning Session

Our team will review your results with you and develop three customized treatment options based on your specific condition, time availability, financial means, goals, and lifestyle. We'll explain each option clearly and answer all your questions.

All of this happens in one day, and on rare occasions, two days. No months of driving back and forth to appointments, insurance delays, and bureaucratic hurdles. Imagine that all in one day! Sounds pretty good, doesn't it?

# WHAT THIS MEANS FOR YOUR FUTURE

My goal with this book isn't to pressure you into anything. It's to give you something the traditional system rarely provides: true clarity about your condition and the confidence to take back control of your future.

Katie's story isn't just about her. It's about you. She faced the same doubts, the same fear of hearing bad news, and the same frustration with being told nothing could be done. And just like you, she wanted her life back. Today, she's hiking again, doing CrossFit, and most importantly, living without the constant fear her body might betray her.

Tom and Linda's story is about you, too. They were tired, overwhelmed, and stuck in a system that gave them more questions than answers. What changed everything was the moment they stopped running from the truth and chose clarity instead. "Not knowing was worse than knowing," Linda told me. And once they understood what they were facing, real decisions and real healing became possible.

*Once you understand what you're facing, real decisions and real healing become possible.*

The same can be true for you. You don't have to keep guessing. You don't have to wait for things to get worse. You don't have to live with fear as your companion.

If you've been waiting for the perfect time to take control of your health, this is it. Not because I say so, but because clarity gives you power, and once you have it, no one can take it away.

Your journey to healing begins with a single decision to finally get the real answers about what's happening in your body. Because once you know the truth, you can chart your own path forward with confidence and hope.

Because the truth is, your story is part of something even bigger: a movement to change the future of joint care forever by creating a world where knee replacement surgery is no longer necessary by 2043.

# CHAPTER 7

# BUT WHAT IF IT DOESN'T WORK FOR ME?

In Chapter 2, you met Wayne, my first patient, when I joined my first practice. But what I didn't share was the rest of Wayne's journey — one that clearly captures why so many people doubt that anything other than surgery will work for them.

Wayne's story isn't about someone who was skeptical of our approach. It's about someone who had been so convinced by the medical system that surgery was his only option that he couldn't imagine any other possibility existed.

If you're reading this chapter thinking, *The Victory Method and knee repair probably won't work for me*, Wayne's story might surprise you. Because Wayne didn't doubt that he needed help to fix his joint, he was skeptical about the possibility that an alternative to surgery could work for him.

## THE SETUP FOR SURGERY

Wayne didn't start out as my patient — he was a patient of the retiring orthopedic surgeon I was replacing. As a result, he'd already been scheduled to have his knee replacement surgery performed by me, as the incoming surgeon.

Wayne had been dealing with knee pain for years, stemming from a football injury in high school back in the 1970s. In those days, when you tore your ACL, orthopedic surgeons performed what Wayne called "the big surgery," which involved cutting the patient wide open and removing their entire meniscus. No arthroscopic meniscus repairs, no partial removals, no attempts to preserve tissue. They just took all the shock-absorbing cartilage (the meniscus) out of the knee and sent you on your way.

More than 20 years later, the inevitable had happened. Without a meniscus cushioning his knee joint, Wayne developed bone-on-bone arthritis in that part of his knee, which stood out plain as day on his x-rays.

Wayne worked as a corrections officer — a demanding job that required him to be on his feet for long shifts, ready to run or handle physical altercations with inmates. The knee pain had become a constant companion, affecting his work performance, his sleep, and life with his wife, Maryann.

When I joined the practice, one of my new partners set clear expectations for Wayne. "We have this new, young surgeon coming in who trained with the greatest orthopedic surgeon of all time, and he will perform your knee replacement surgery," they told him.

Wayne was ready. Actually, he was excited. After years of pain, cortisone shots that stopped working after a while, and watching his function decline, he was finally going to get his knee fixed. He came to that first appointment expecting to discuss the details of his upcoming operation so he could get on with the process of recovery.

## THE UNEXPECTED CONVERSATION

After I examined his knee thoroughly, I spent time looking at his x-rays — really studying them, not just giving them a quick glance and confirming what everyone already knew. I asked detailed questions about his symptoms, his work demands, and his goals beyond getting rid of the pain.

And then I said something Wayne wasn't expecting: "You don't need a knee replacement."

The air seemed to go out of the room as I watched confusion wash over his face. Here was a 43-year-old man who had been told by multiple doctors that surgery was inevitable, who had psyched himself up for the procedure, who was ready to finally get this over with, and suddenly, the surgeon who was supposed to fix him was telling him the opposite.

"What do you mean?" Wayne replied. "Look at these x-rays. It's bone-on-bone. Everyone's told me this needs to be replaced."

Maybe you're feeling the same way Wayne did. Maybe you've been told your painful joint is bone-on-bone, or that replacement is your only option. But it isn't, and here's why.

I pulled out my flip chart — the same anatomical diagrams I'd been using since my fellowship days — and showed Wayne something no doctor had ever taken the time to explain: How his knee actually worked, what had happened when they removed his meniscus all those years ago, and why his cartilage had worn down in that predictable pattern.

Most importantly, I explained why being only 43 made all the difference in the world.

"Wayne, knee replacements wear out. On average, they last 15 to 20 years. If we put metal, plastic, and cement in your knee now, you'll likely need another surgery when you're in your early sixties," I said.

After a quick pause to make sure he was understanding me, I added, "Revision surgeries are much more complicated, don't last as long, and don't work as well as first-time replacements. If we can get you to retirement age without surgery, wouldn't that be worth trying?"

Wayne stared at the diagram, then back at his x-rays. "What exactly are you proposing?" he asked.

I outlined a different approach. This was 1998, so I didn't yet have access to many of the regenerative treatments we use today, but I had the foundational principles I'd learned during my fellowship with Dr. Andrews. I'd exhaust every nonoperative option before considering surgery, treat the whole person rather than just the joint, and never underestimate the body's ability to adapt and heal when given the right support.

Wayne listened, but I could tell he was more bewildered than convinced. He had come in expecting one conversation and was getting an entirely different one.

"Look," he finally said, "I'll try it. But I have to be honest, I was ready to get this surgery done. I don't really understand how this other stuff is going to help when the cartilage is already gone."

I understood his confusion, just as I understand yours. The entire medical system had conditioned him to think in terms of damaged parts that needed to be replaced, not as a person whose body might still have healing potential.

"Give me three months," I said. "If you're not significantly better, we can always revisit the surgery option. But let's see what's possible first."

Wayne agreed, though I could tell he was mostly going through the motions to be polite to the new doctor who was supposed to have been his surgeon. Or at least, that's what I thought.

## THE REAL TESTIMONY

A few days after Wayne's appointment, I'd just sat down in the recovery area to finish dictating my operative report after a surgery when one of the nurses approached me.

"Excuse me, Dr. Pietropaoli?" she said.

"Yes?"

"I'm Maryann. Wayne's wife."

My heart skipped a beat. I wasn't sure how Wayne had processed our conversation, and I was nervous about what his wife might say. Had he gone home frustrated? Angry that the new doctor was trying to talk him out of the surgery he'd been promised?

"I just wanted to thank you," she said.

I was surprised. "Thank me for what?"

"For telling him he doesn't need surgery."

"He was so relieved," she continued, and I could hear the genuine emotion in her voice.

"I wasn't sure how he took that news, to be honest," I confessed.

"He couldn't believe it. You know, I've been telling him all along that he didn't need a knee replacement — at least not yet. I work in the recovery room here. I see what happens with these surgeries every day. It's not always the best solution, and there can be complications. But Wayne wouldn't listen to me. When you told him the same thing, he was amazed. And I was so grateful."

She went on to explain that Wayne had been much more worried about the surgery than he'd let on. The recovery time, the limitations, the possibility of complications, and the effect on his work — all of it had been weighing on him heavily.

"He was excited about finally getting it over with," Maryann said, "but he was also scared. When you told him there might be another way, it was like a huge weight lifted off his shoulders."

Then she said something that has stayed with me for more than 25 years: "You don't get too many surgeons who tell people they *don't* need surgery. Certainly not around here. Wayne was super impressed with you."

Right there in that recovery room, I realized something crucial. Wayne's apparent confusion during our appointment wasn't skepticism about whether the treatment would work; it was disbelief that he had an option other than surgery. He had been so conditioned to believe that bone-on-bone equals immediate knee replacement that the possibility of alternatives had never even occurred to him.

Like Wayne, you may feel conditioned to believe your body has no healing potential. But Wayne's story proves otherwise, and so can yours.

More than that, Maryann's words showed me something I've seen consistently over the past 27 years: Even when patients say they're ready for surgery, even when they seem eager to get it over with, there's often

> *Even when patients say they're ready for surgery, even when they seem eager to get it over with, there's often an underlying fear that surgery isn't the best option and a hope that maybe there's another way.*

an underlying fear that surgery isn't the best option and a hope that maybe there's another way.

## THE LONG GAME PAYOFF

Ultimately, Wayne didn't have his knee replacement until he was 66, 23 years after his first appointment with me.

Let that sink in for a moment. 23 years.

Wayne eventually moved away to Florida, and by the time he was persuaded to have his knee replaced, he was retired and could afford the recovery time.

He'd lived more than two decades of active life without the limitations, restrictions, and risks that can come with artificial joints. He'd worked his entire career without missing time for major surgery. He'd maintained his independence, his mobility, and his quality of life well into his 60s.

Most importantly, he never needed the complex revision surgery that often becomes necessary when younger people have joint replacements in their 40s and 50s and the initial artificial joint wears out.

## WHAT THE DATA SHOWS NOW

Our capabilities have evolved exponentially since 1998. Back when I initially treated Wayne, I was prescribing physical therapy, activity modification, and the foundational principles from my fellowship. Today, we have regenerative medicine treatments that can actually *repair* damaged tissue at the cellular level. We have bone marrow stem cells and other cells that help the stem cells restore and heal cartilage and bone. We also have advanced laser therapy that supports healing at the mitochondrial level. And we have precision imaging that guides exact treatment protocols.

If Wayne was able to delay surgery for 23 years with the help of 1998 technology and treatments, imagine what's possible now.

In 2022, we reviewed our own patients' results and found that 91 percent of those who completed our comprehensive programs achieved their personal goals without surgery. These aren't carefully selected patients with minor problems; they are people like Wayne and people like you who are middle-aged or older, arthritic, experiencing increasing pain, and told by multiple doctors that replacement was inevitable.

## WHEN DOUBT CREEPS IN

Let me share the most common fears joint sufferers express, because I've heard them thousands of times and I experienced some myself, if you recall my story from Chapter 4. You might recognize yourself in one of these doubts. Maybe you've thought, *My damage is too severe*, *I've already tried everything*, or, *I can't afford it*. If so, you're not alone.

### "My damage looks too severe."

I think about Sarah, a 52-year-old teacher whose x-rays looked worse than Wayne's. Three orthopedic surgeons had told her she needed bilateral knee replacements, and she came to me as a last resort, certain I'd say the same thing.

Instead, we addressed the underlying bone health, strengthened and rebuilt her supporting muscles, and used regenerative medicine treatments to improve her joint function. Two years later, she's hiking with her husband and has never had surgery.

If you've been shown an x-ray or MRI that seems to be proof positive your joint is too far gone, *of course* you're going to believe you have only one option. But as you've seen from the patient stories in this book, there are always other possible choices — and other outcomes.

## "I've already tried everything."

That's what Jim told me. He'd been through traditional physical therapy three times, had multiple cortisone shots, tried gel injections, and even considered experimental treatments overseas. But he'd never had anyone look at his whole-body system or address the inflammation that was preventing healing.

Once we optimized his nutrition, fixed his sleep cycle that was affecting recovery, and used regenerative and functional medicine treatments, his pain dropped from an eight on a scale of 10, to a two *within six months.*

If you've reached the point of giving up on alternatives because of all the treatments you've already been through, the question to ask yourself is not, "Have I tried enough?" It's "Did any of those attempts truly look at my condition holistically and get to the *root cause* of my pain and how my body can heal?"

## "I'm running out of time."

Jennifer was 48 when she came to see me, convinced she was too young for replacement but too old for healing. Her surgeon had told her to "Suck it up and wait until you can't stand it anymore. Then come back and see me." Sound familiar?

When we started her Victory Method program, she discovered that her body was more resilient than anyone had given it credit for. She's now 55, more active than she was at 40, and has never needed surgery.

If you, like Jennifer, think you're simply too old to heal, if you're alive enough to read this book, you've still got time.

## "We can't afford this."

Janise came to us with her husband, Taras, after injuring her knee on a cruise. She'd been told she needed a total knee replacement and came to us for other options.

For years, she and Taras had been saving up to travel, but now could not enjoy those retirement funds due to her knee pain. Both were very interested in Knee Repair, NOT Knee Replacement but Janise was hesitant to proceed due to the cost.

Taras had been silent for most of the initial appointment but started squirming in his chair more and more as his wife hemmed and hawed about proceeding. Finally, he spoke up.

"Honey, I can't sleep at night because you're always moaning in pain. This is affecting me too. What good is our retirement money if we can't enjoy it? This is an investment, not a cost, in your — in *our* — future So let's just do it!" he said.

Twelve weeks later, at Janise's follow-up appointment, Taras came up to me, misty eyed, and said, "You gave me my wife back. You gave us our *lives* back."

I recently got a postcard from the two of them that said, "Now we're on a tour of the southern US!"

The process I've been describing is not a small investment, and money is a serious, legitimate concern when you're weighing your personal situation, your deepest feelings, and treatment options. But to arrive at the best decision, factor in all the costs involved in whatever path you choose.

Not just the direct cost of surgery versus joint repair, but the cost in time away from work, physical and emotional pain, risk of complications, and the need for a second, revision replacement in the future. Most of all, the cost of giving up on a life and a future you dreamed of.

## "I could waste months trying this if it does not work."

This was exactly Wayne's concern. While it is true the treatment or program may not work to your satisfaction, the odds are with you at least an 82-95 percent success rate, and at the time of writing of this book, a 94 percent satisfaction rate.

Still, it's important to remember that no treatment is 100 percent successful, not even surgery. Most surgeries are considered successful if they have an 80-95 percent success rate. The only things in life that are 100 percent are death and taxes, so what if this doesn't work? Consider this: Even if you eventually need surgery, optimizing your health, your strength, your range of motion, your muscle mass, and your mechanics first makes that surgery safer and more successful.

> *Even if you eventually need surgery, optimizing your health, your strength, your range of motion, your muscle mass, and your mechanics first makes that surgery safer and more successful.*

Patients who come to surgery healthier, stronger, and less inflamed recover faster and have better outcomes. There's no downside to becoming healthier before any major procedure. Our goal is to prevent you from needing surgery if we can, but if you do need it, you have not wasted your time.

## "Mom will never commit to doing this."

Pat came to me as a last resort at the request of her family. She was 86 years old and had knee, hip, and back pain so severe, she was considering moving out of the home she had lived in for decades.

"I would hate to move from the home where I've shared so many wonderful memories with my family. I'd consider your program, Marc, but my family doesn't think I'd commit to the process — or even be able to get through it."

Oftentimes, it's not the patient who's the impediment to healing, it's the patient's family. When I first saw and evaluated Pat, she was using a walker and could not get out of a chair on her own. But she ignored her family's judgment, doubts, and objections, and twelve weeks after undergoing one of our best comprehensive programs, she easily got up out of that same chair with a smile. With tears in her eyes, she gave me a huge hug.

Pat was able to remain in the home she loved and avoided losing her independence. "She proved us all wrong," her daughter, Carol, later told me. "She is doing things we haven't seen her do since her condition began."

You may be reading this book because you have a loved one who is facing the prospect of a knee replacement, and you worry they won't be capable of going through the process I've been outlining.

Or perhaps you have joint pain of your own, and you're excited about the possibility of repairing your joint, not replacing it, but you're struggling with family and friends who are doubtful and discouraging you from taking an alternative approach to surgery.

If so, just remember the unexpected power that comes as you feel your body healing itself within days of starting treatment. And give your loved one — or yourself — the opportunity to stand up for their choice.

## "It will be too painful"

I am not going to include a single story here, because *every* patient worries about this — even *I* worried about this when I had my elbow repaired. Patients are particularly afraid of the bone marrow harvesting part of the process. But while it sounds scary and painful, I recently asked 10 patients in a row who underwent bone marrow harvest to obtain the stem cells and other cells that help the stem cells about the experience, and 10 out of 10 said, "It wasn't that bad," or "It wasn't as bad as I thought it was going to be."

It's true that everyone handles pain and procedures differently, but speaking for myself, the pain from my regenerative medicine procedure was there, but was nowhere near the pain I'd experienced during five previous surgeries. The vast majority of our patients feel the same way.

## "None of my other doctors ever told me about this, so it couldn't be that good or it's too risky"

The truth is that most doctors and medical providers are not versed on biologic, regenerative medicine, or on other holistic and natural ways of treating patients. It's not their fault. They simply aren't trained on these techniques by the traditional medical system.

So, if you've encountered doctors with this bias, just ask them for *concrete, high-level research and data* that proves surgery is the only option, and that these alternative treatments don't work.

## THE SYSTEM'S BUILT-IN BIAS

Wayne's case revealed something important about our health-care system. He had been programmed — by doctors, by his insurance company, by the entire medical establishment — to see his situation through a hammer-nail surgical lens. Here's the typical conversation:

Patient:   "My knee hurts."
Doctor:   "Your x-ray shows arthritis. You'll eventually need a replacement."
Patient:   "Is there anything else we can try?"
Doctor:   "We can do some shots or physical therapy to buy you time, but ultimately you'll need surgery."

This creates a self-fulfilling prophecy. When your only tool is a hammer, everything looks like a nail. When doctors are trained primarily in surgical solutions, every joint problem looks like it needs surgery.

> *When your only tool is a hammer, everything looks like a nail. When doctors are trained primarily in surgical solutions, every joint problem looks like it needs surgery.*

But joints aren't just mechanical structures, they're part of living, adaptable, healable human bodies. Wayne's story proves that what multiple doctors called "necessary" wasn't needed at that time.

## WHAT THIS MEANS FOR YOU

Wayne came to me expecting surgery and left with hope. He came into my office resigned to his fate and discovered he had choices. Most importantly, he learned that what multiple doctors had told him was his only choice, was not his only choice at all.

I'm not asking you to believe our approach will work for you. I'm asking whether you're open to discovering that *you might have options you didn't know existed.*

Wayne would tell you now, "Don't assume you know all your options just because that's what you've been told. I almost had surgery I didn't need 23 years too early. The best decision I ever made was listening to Dr. P when he said there might be another way."

Wayne trusted the possibilities and the data enough to postpone surgery for three months so he could see what was possible. That three-month delay turned into 23 years of active life with his original joints.

What if the same thing is true for you?

What if this time, you discovered you had choices you didn't know existed?

What if the surgery you think you need is actually the surgery you can avoid?

Sometimes the best treatment is avoiding the surgery you don't have to have.

Sometimes curiosity is just skepticism with an open mind.

And sometimes, what everyone tells you is inevitable, isn't.

# CHAPTER 8

# TIME, MONEY, AND REAL LIFE

I've been doing this for more than thirty years, and I can predict the exact moment when someone's face changes during our conversation. It happens right after they start believing that, yes, maybe their knee really can be repaired. Maybe they don't need surgery after all. Maybe there is hope.

But that's when their other beliefs and fears appear.

"But Dr. P," they say, "I don't have time for a three-month program."

Sometimes they say, "It sounds great, but we can't afford this right now."

Or my personal favorite: "My spouse, children, family, and coworkers think I should just get the knee replacement and be done with it."

I get it. I really do. These are real concerns from real people living real lives. You're not making excuses, you're being practical. But what I've

*What I've learned after helping more than 30,000 people repair their joints is that the biggest risk isn't making your health a priority; your biggest risk is waiting until you have no other choices left.*

learned after helping more than 30,000 people repair their joints is that the biggest risk isn't making your health a priority; your biggest risk is waiting until you have no other choices left.

## THE REAL-TIME MATH

Here's what actually happens when you go through the traditional system versus a holistic process.

One day, you wake up with knee pain and call your primary care doctor. They can schedule you for an appointment in two weeks, and when you arrive, you'll sit in the waiting room for 45 minutes, only to spend seven minutes with the doctor.

Their advice? Try ibuprofen and come back in three months.

Three months later, you're back. Another wait, another quick visit. "Let's get some x-rays," your doctor says. "You'll have to call the imaging center down the road to set up the appointment."

Several days later, you drive to the imaging center, and your x-rays are performed, but when you ask what your x-rays show, you're told, "Your doctor will have to call you with the results."

Two weeks later, your doctor still hasn't called you with the results, so you call your doctor's office, and they act surprised that you're even asking. "We can't give you the results," they'll say. "Your doctor will have to call you. We'll let her know, and she'll call you back with the results."

Three days later — still in pain — your doctor calls you back. You hear her typing on the computer as she says, "The report says you have osteoarthritis. You'll probably need a knee replacement, but let's try physical therapy first. We will have to get authorization from your insurance company."

Three weeks later, the insurance finally authorizes your physical therapy. Your primary care office calls and tells you where they referred you to, but that you'll have to call them and set up your appointments.

When you finally get ahold of the physical therapist's office, they tell you they can see you, but not for another two weeks.

After six weeks of therapy, twice a week, you've had 12 appointments — 12 drives back and forth and 12 co-pays. Sure, maybe it helps a little, but you're still in pain.

"Now we can order an MRI?" you ask your doctor. That's when you find out the average wait time for an MRI in the US is two to four weeks.

How long have you been dealing with this now? Six months? A year? Most of my patients have been stuck in this cycle for years.

Now compare the traditional approach to The Victory Method Clarity Day.

## THE CYCLE OF INSANITY
### Knee Pain and the Healthcare System

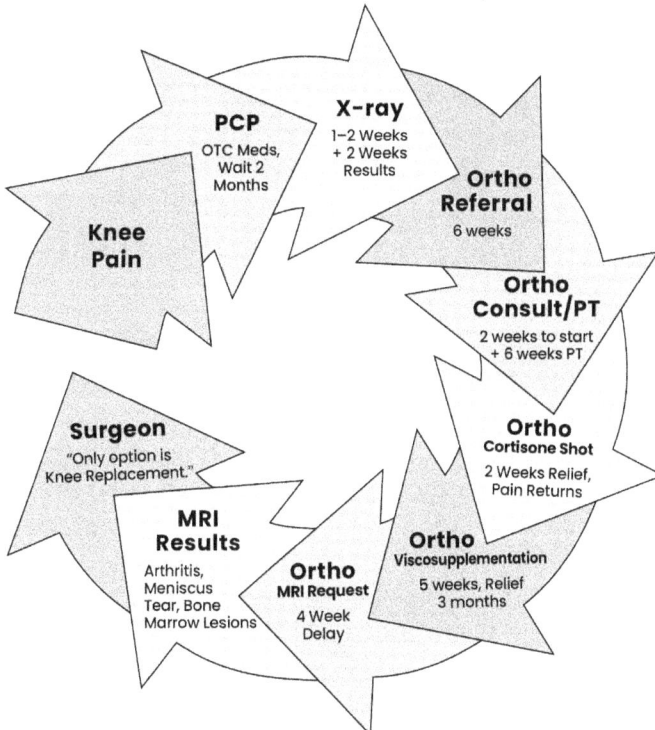

**PCP**
OTC Meds, Wait 2 Months

**X-ray**
1–2 Weeks + 2 Weeks Results

**Knee Pain**

**Ortho Referral**
6 weeks

**Ortho Consult/PT**
2 weeks to start + 6 weeks PT

**Ortho** Cortisone Shot
2 Weeks Relief, Pain Returns

**Ortho** Viscosupplementation
5 weeks, Relief 3 months

**Surgeon**
"Only option is Knee Replacement."

**MRI Results**
Arthritis, Meniscus Tear, Bone Marrow Lesions

**Ortho** MRI Request
4 Week Delay

**Total Time: ~54 Weeks**

## CLARITY DAY™
### Knee Pain and the Victory In Motion Team Experience

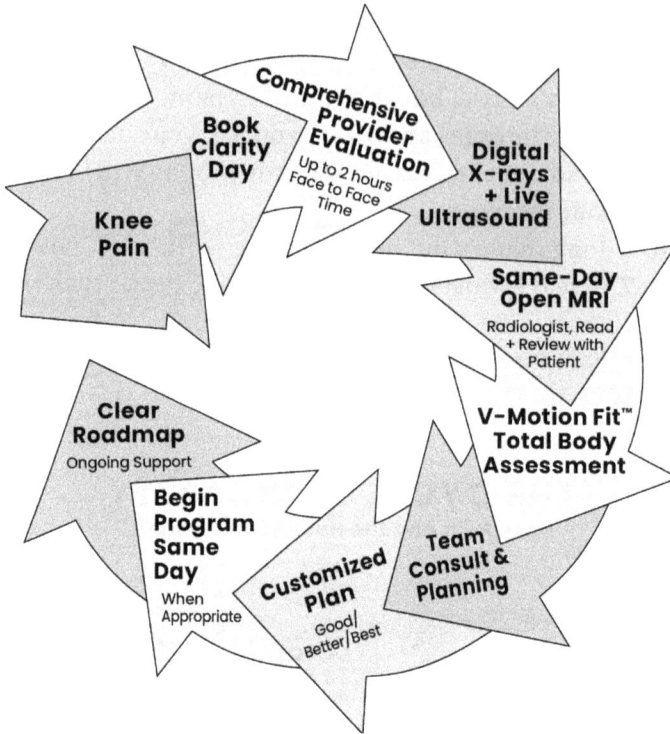

Knee Pain

Book Clarity Day

Comprehensive Provider Evaluation
Up to 2 hours Face to Face Time

Digital X-rays + Live Ultrasound

Same-Day Open MRI
Radiologist, Read + Review with Patient

V-Motion Fit™ Total Body Assessment

Team Consult & Planning

Customized Plan
Good/Better/Best

Begin Program Same Day
When Appropriate

Clear Roadmap
Ongoing Support

**Total Time: 1 Day**

Four to five hours. One visit. 60-minute consultation, digital x-rays with immediate review, live ultrasound evaluation, specialized open MRI with same-day results and review, complete whole-body strength assessment, and a clear diagnosis with customized treatment plan.

And if you do choose surgery? The recovery time is almost always much longer with surgery than with a non-operative regenerative medicine procedure and program.

So...which approach actually saves you time?

The unfortunate truth is that every day you wait to make a decision about the right treatment path for you, your joint can deteriorate a little more. The stress/microfractures in the bone can spread. The inflammation usually increases. The surrounding muscles can weaken from compensation patterns. And once you develop those microfractures or soft spots, research shows you're nine times more likely to need a knee replacement.[21]

Time isn't neutral when it comes to joint and musculoskeletal health. Time is working against you.

*Time isn't neutral when it comes to joint and musculoskeletal health. Time is working against you.*

When people tell me they don't have time to fix their knee, I ask them: "How much time are you spending managing your pain right now?"

Think about it. How much time do you spend researching pain relief options online on YouTube, Facebook, Instagram, or even TikTok? So many people have so many thoughts and opinions, but there's no real clarity.

Trying different sleeping positions? Shopping for braces and pain creams? Planning activities around your limitations? Explaining to your family why you can't do certain things? Worrying about whether you'll need surgery eventually? That takes time too. Wasted time, if I might say. It's time spent managing a problem instead of solving it.

Now let's talk about what you've probably been wondering since you began Chapter 1: *How much will this investment in my health cost?*

I'm not going to sugarcoat this. The comprehensive Victory Method programs require a significant investment. Why? Because insurance companies don't cover treatments that allow your body to heal itself.

It's not your fault; it's not our fault; it's not the doctors' fault. It's the fault of the medical system and the insurance companies that back it up. There are a lot of special interests that do not want the system to change. They cannot regulate how your body produces platelets, growth factors, or stem cells, so, naturally, they don't want us using your own naturally occurring body parts. Instead, they'd rather you use factory-manufactured, artificial parts.

I recently had a patient say, "Doc, I cannot thank you enough for healing me. I am so, so appreciative."

I said, "I did not heal you; *you* healed you. I harvested your cells and blood growth factors, concentrated them, and using ultrasonic guidance, injected them precisely where your body needed these healing cells and growth factors. Then *you* healed yourself! Congratulations, and thank *you!*"

When prospective patients facing long, painful joint replacement hear the cost of investing in a faster, less painful, and more effective alternative, I usually see their faces change from hope to disappointment.

But let me share even more of Tom's story, because it changed how I think about this conversation.

Tom came to us weighing 368 pounds and spent $300–400 a month on medications for blood pressure, cholesterol, and diabetes. His doctor had told him that without major lifestyle changes, he'd likely need more medications and eventually, joint replacements in both knees and possibly his hips.

"Dr. P," Tom said during our consultation, "my wife and I have been saving for our retirement. We want to travel, see our kids, and enjoy our grandchildren. But honestly, at this rate, I'm not going to be healthy enough to enjoy any of it."

Tom invested in one of our wellness optimization programs we designed specifically for him. Within six months, his primary care doctor had taken him off all three of his medications. All of them. Does that happen for everyone? No. But it does happen for many people just like Tom and just like you and me.

Let's crunch Tom's actual numbers. At $350 per month in medications, he was spending $4,200 per year. Over his remaining 20-year life expectancy, that's $84,000 in medications alone. That doesn't include doctor visits, lab work, or the eventual joint surgeries his doctor predicted he'd need.

During his follow-up visit, Tom's emotions were clear when he said, "Dr. P, you didn't just save me money, you gave me back my future. My wife and I are planning that trip to Italy we've talked about for years. Six months ago, I couldn't walk to the mailbox without getting winded. Last week, I walked five miles."

Tom's investment in the program? Less than what he would have spent on medications in two years.

## WHAT MY FATHER TAUGHT ME

I think about my dad often when patients express concern about the cost of treatment. Dad was a practical man. He worked in construction to put himself through college and law school, and he knew the value of a dollar and the importance of making smart investments.

When Dad needed his hip replacement, I tried to convince him to explore other options first. But he was focused on what seemed like the economical choice. "Insurance covers the surgery," he said. "Why would I pay out of pocket for something else?"

What Dad didn't factor in was the cost of complications. Nine years after his replacement, it became infected. The surgery to remove it left him with a shortened leg and months in rehabilitation. The stress contributed to other health problems. In the end, the total financial and emotional cost was far more than any preventive approach would have been.

"Son," he told me while I was changing the dressing on his huge hip wound, "I wish I'd listened to you about trying other options first. I thought I was being smart with money, but I was being foolish with my health."

## THE REAL QUESTION YOU NEED TO ASK

When patients express concern about the investment, I ask them one question: "What would it be worth to you to avoid a knee replacement?"

Just the surgery itself costs $30,000–50,000. Depending on your insurance, you could be responsible for a significant portion of that amount — especially if you have a high-deductible plan. But that's just the beginning.

You'll need to factor in time off work (four to six weeks minimum on average), months of physical therapy, potential complications, the limitations that come with artificial joints, and the fact that replacements typically require a revision surgery every 10–20 years, depending on your age and activity level.

When you factor in the lifetime costs, knee replacement becomes far more expensive than repair.

But beyond the financial costs, what about the costs you can't measure in dollars?

What's it worth to sleep through the night without pain? To get down on the floor and play with your grandchildren without limitation? To travel without worrying about stairs or walking distances? To feel confident and stable on your feet again?

*What's it worth to sleep through the night without pain? To get down on the floor and play with your grandchildren without limitation? To travel without worrying about stairs or walking distances? To feel confident and stable on your feet again?*

## WHEN FAMILIES DON'T UNDERSTAND

One of the most challenging conversations I have is when patients say, "My family thinks I should just get the surgery and be done with it."

I understand this completely. When you're in pain, everyone wants to help. And to someone who isn't living in your body every day, surgery can seem like the quick fix. But here's what I've observed in my thirty years of practice: The family member who pressures their loved one to get the surgery is often the same person who becomes the caregiver during the difficult recovery period.

They're the ones helping with daily activities for weeks. They're the ones driving to multiple physical therapy appointments. They're the ones watching their loved ones struggle with the limitations that come with artificial joints. And they're the ones shouldering the worry when complications arise for the person they love.

The part that breaks my heart is they're also often the ones who say, months later, "I wish we'd known there was another option."

But when The Victory Method works, the benefits aren't just for you. Your whole family gets you back.

I had one patient's husband tell me through tears, "You didn't just give my wife her life back. *You gave us our lives back. Now* we're planning the retirement travel we used to think was impossible."

## MAKING IT WORK

I know people have different financial situations, family dynamics, and life circumstances, but the truth is that when something matters enough, we find a way to make it happen.

Think about it this way: By mid-2025, the average new car in the United States cost roughly $48,800, and the average used car hovered around $25,200.[22] Most of us don't blink an eye at those numbers. We maintain our cars, insure them, and replace them every few years, yet we only spend about an hour a day actually using them.

Now, compare that to your body. You live in it 24 hours a day, seven days a week, 365 days a year. And yet, when it comes to investing in the body that carries you through every moment of your life, you hesitate.

So, let me ask you:

- What costs more: Acting now while you have options, or waiting until replacement is your only choice?
- What costs more: Three months of focused healing, or years of gradual decline?
- What costs more: Investing in your health today, or managing pain for the rest of your life?

Health is not an expense. Health is an investment that pays dividends every single day for the rest of your life.

I've had patients tell me they regretted waiting. I've had patients tell me they wished they'd found us sooner. I've even had patients who regretted having surgery to replace their joints. But I've never once had someone tell me they regretted doing everything they could to invest in their health.

*Health is not an expense. Health is an investment that pays dividends every single day for the rest of your life.*

So, if you've been hesitating because of time, money, or family pressures, remember that the cost of waiting is always higher than the cost of acting.

The only real question left is: *What are you waiting for?*

# CHAPTER 9

# STRONGER, LONGER: HOW TO STAY IN MOTION

It wasn't the first time Pam had fallen. At 71, working at Syracuse University with the young people she loved, she'd grown accustomed to the occasional stumble — moments when her knees would give out without warning. But this time was different. This time, she'd hit the ground hard.

By the time her x-rays came back, her son, Josh, had joined her in the emergency room.

"I'm afraid you have a fractured pelvis," the doctor told them.

Pam looked at her son, the weight of another injury settling over her like a heavy blanket.

"You know what this means," she said quietly. "I'm going to lose all my independence."

"No, Mom," Josh replied firmly. "We'll do whatever it takes to make sure that doesn't happen."

The fractured pelvis was devastating, but the real problem was that her knees had been failing her for years. The repeated falls, the fear, the gradual loss of activities she loved — it was all connected to her deteriorating knees.

Before her problems began, Pam had been active and independent. She worked full-time, traveled, and took pride in maintaining her home and garden. But over the past few years, simple activities had become mountains to climb. Getting up from chairs required planning and assistance. Stairs had become enemies. Even walking to her car felt uncertain and dangerous. For someone who thrived on working with students and maintaining her independence, this progressive decline felt like watching her life disappear piece by piece.

But there was one specific moment that crystallized things for Pam. An important award ceremony was coming up at Syracuse University in recognition of her years of dedicated service working with young people. It should have been a celebration, but instead, it had become a source of dread.

"If I could just get up from a chair without fear of falling," she told Josh, "especially at that award ceremony coming up, I'd feel like I had my life back. I won't even be able to go now."

That ceremony represented everything she was losing: her dignity, her confidence, and her ability to participate in the work community that meant so much to her.

When doctors inevitably recommended knee replacement surgery, Pam's response was immediate and definitive. "No," she said. "I'm never going to do that."

She'd watched too many friends struggle with knee replacements and had seen the limitations, complications, and ongoing issues. The idea terrified her more than living with the pain.

Fortunately, most pelvis fractures from falls don't require surgery and can heal with rehabilitation, physical therapy, and time. But as her pelvis healed, the underlying problem remained. Her knees were still failing her, and her fear of falling was still controlling her life.

But Josh wouldn't let her give up. "Don't worry, Mom. We'll figure something out."

That's when they found Victory In Motion.

## A DIFFERENT PATH

When Pam came into my office for her comprehensive evaluation, she already knew us because we'd helped with her pelvis recovery. But this time was different — this time we were addressing the root cause of her falls.

As soon as she met with Allison, our orthopedic physician assistant, she knew The Victory Method was different. Allison listened and understood her goals. Then, the team reviewed her full history and examined her knees with ultrasound imaging.

The MRI showed stress and microfracturing in the bone underneath the cartilage in her knee. Because bone contains millions of pressure-sensitive nerve fibers, these soft spots were causing Pam an immense amount of pain.

"We can help you avoid knee replacement surgery," Allison and I told her. "But it's going to require a comprehensive approach."

Pam began with the same regenerative medicine procedure that Katie and Randi experienced. Using her own bone marrow aspirate, which contains stem cells and other healing cells and platelet-rich plasma, her bones and body began healing themselves.

For the first time in years, Pam felt true hope.

Now she was ready to begin working with our V-Motion Fit team. As we talked about the next steps in her journey, I could hear a new degree of nervousness and uncertainty in her voice.

"Don't worry," I told her. "We'll guide you at your own pace. I think you'll be amazed at what you'll be capable of doing."

Our V-Motion Fit team met Pam where she was, both physically and emotionally. They told her that recovery was 20 percent physical and 80 percent mental. They created an individualized total-body plan that built both mental and physical confidence and strength, retraining her balance, mechanics and movement patterns.

Before long, Pam was doing exercises like weighted deadlifts and squats that she never thought she'd be doing at her age. They made her feel stronger and more confident, and they reduced the fear of falling that had been consuming her.

The team also taught her that her back, along with the tightness in her ankle tendons and hip, was affecting her knee — crucial pieces of information she hadn't understood before.

As they worked on her body in a holistic manner, it all started to make sense. "It's like that old song, *Dem Bones*," Pam told them with a smile. "The knee bone connected to the thigh bone, the thigh bone connected to the hip bone. I remember that from when I was a kid."

She worked out two to three times a week, building strength and confidence. But one day, she overdid her deadlifts and had a setback. Her knee buckled, and for a moment she was devastated, thinking she was back at square one and worried she might fall again.

But her team helped her understand this wasn't unusual; she just needed to continue working on strengthening her quadriceps and all her muscles. After a couple more V-Motion Fit visits, the buckling never happened again.

## THE MOMENT OF TRUTH

The real test came six months later at the award ceremony, where Pam was being recognized for her years of service working with young people, something that had given her life so much meaning.

As she sat in the audience, waiting for her name to be called, she felt a familiar flutter of anxiety. But this time, it wasn't the paralyzing fear she'd lived with for years. This time, she felt confident.

When they announced her name, Pam stood up from her chair — without a cane, without fear, without hesitation. She walked up the stairs to the stage, received her award, and felt a pride that went far beyond the recognition itself. She had conquered her fear of falling. She was in control of her body again.

The contrast was striking. The day we first saw her, she couldn't stand up from a chair without assistance, and she was terrified of falling. Now she was walking confidently across a stage in front of hundreds of people who were all celebrating her achievements.

## THE SCIENCE OF STAYING STRONG

What Pam discovered — and what research consistently shows — is that successful joint repair is just the beginning. The real key to long-term success is maintaining the strength, mobility, and function you've regained.

Studies show that adults lose three to eight percent of their muscle mass per decade after age 30, and this loss accelerates after age 65.[23] For people with joint problems, this muscle loss is often even more pronounced due to reduced activity and compensation patterns.

The encouraging part is that research also shows that resistance training can not only slow this decline but can actually reverse it. Published scientific literature shows that adults older than 65 who engaged in regular strength training actually increased their muscle mass and improved their bone density.[24]

For joint health specifically, maintaining strong supporting muscles is crucial. The quadriceps and all the other muscles of the lower extremities act as shock absorbers for the knee joint. When those muscles are weak, more force is transmitted directly to the joint surfaces, accelerating wear and potentially undermining whatever repair work has been accomplished.

This is why our maintenance approach isn't optional; it's essential for protecting your hard work and investment in healing.

## BEYOND RECOVERY: TWO PATHS TO SUCCESS

Pam and Diane show us that there is more than one way forward after joint repair. As I shared in Chapter 5, there are at least two post-treatment paths, and the right one for you depends on your lifestyle and goals.

Pam is one of our "60+ Golden VIP Girls." They are the fastest growing group of V-Motion Fit participants we have. She didn't just recover, she got stronger, more confident, and more capable than she'd been in years. Her path is what we call **Supported Maintenance**.

Her routine is simple but consistent: She comes into our office one to three times a week, and we adjust her program as needed. Are you someone who likes accountability, structure, and guidance? So does Pam, and that is why she — and you — will be most successful in Supported Maintenance.

Fortunately, if you live too far to commute regularly to our clinic, Supported Maintenance can still be possible for you through telecommunication, video V-Motion Fit sessions. Since COVID-19, we've become true experts at this approach, and many patients actually find it more helpful than in-office visits. Why? Because we get to see you in your element, so to speak. We get to see your home, your gym, or wherever you normally work out. That allows us to design and refine your program with precision, tailored to your exact surroundings, equipment, and routines.

The result is a plan that's not just personalized, but sustainable for the long term. Live in another state? Canada? Europe? Asia? We provide telecommunication, video V-Motion Fit strength and conditioning services, no matter where you are.

Diane's story shows another path. At 79, she was told she needed a knee replacement. After completing her Knee Repair, NOT Knee Replacement Victory Method program, she got her independence back. But instead of regular check-ins, she chose **Independent Maintenance**.

She comes into our office just once a year. On her own, she does yoga daily, walks her dog, and has even added light weights into her routine at the gym. Are you more independent, disciplined, and self-directed? Maybe you like to work out at hours that are not regular workday hours? Independent Maintenance works for Diane, and it can work for you too.

Some people thrive with ongoing professional support, while others prefer independence with occasional guidance. No matter your preference, we have the resources for you. What matters is that you choose the style that fits your personality, your schedule, and your goals.

## THE LONG-TERM REALITY

Here's what both Pam and Diane understand, and what you need to remember: Joint repair isn't a one-time fix. Just like your car, your teeth, your garden, or your mind, your joints need ongoing care.

*Joint repair isn't a one-time fix. Just like your car, your teeth, your garden, or your mind, your joints need ongoing care.*

But unlike managing a joint replacement — with its restrictions, limitations, and risk of revision surgery — maintenance after repair gives you freedom. With the right habits, you don't just hold on to your results; you can keep improving year after year.

### What Maintenance Really Means

Successful maintenance always comes down to three universal principles you can follow whether you're with us in person, connecting by video telecommunication, or applying them on your own:

1. **Consistent Movement:** Whether it's V-Motion Fit, yoga, weight training, or simply walking, your body needs regular resistance and mobility work. Movement is medicine — we *are* Victory In Motion!
2. **Professional Support:** Decide how much guidance you need. Are you like Pam, who thrives with frequent accountability? Or more like Diane, who checks in once a year? With televideo visits, we can meet you where you are and guide you directly in your own space.
3. **Long-Term Perspective:** Maintenance is not a burden; it's self-care that preserves your independence and quality of life.

Still think a long-term maintenance plan is optional? Research shows that people who maintain consistent movement and strength training after repair don't just preserve their results, they often keep improving, even into their 70s, 80s, and 90s.[25]

Does this make sense? Does this sound good to you? Great, keep reading.

## THE CHOICE IS YOURS

The patients who struggle are the ones who treat joint repair like a quick fix and slide back into old habits. The ones who thrive are those who recognize that joint repair gives you the foundation, but you're the one who builds the future on top of it.

Pam said it best: "Dr. P, you didn't just fix my knees. You taught me how to take

> *The patients who struggle are the ones who treat joint repair like a quick fix and slide back into old habits. The ones who thrive are those who recognize that joint repair gives you the foundation, but you're the one who builds the future on top of it.*

care of my whole body. I feel like I have the tools now to age successfully, not just survive getting older."

That's what maintenance really offers you. It's not just preserved joint function, but the ability to age with strength, confidence, and independence. So let me ask you:

- Do you see yourself as someone who will benefit from supported guidance, like Pam — whether in-person or through telecommunication video visits?
- Or do you see yourself thriving with a more independent path, like Diane?

The question isn't whether you'll need maintenance — you will. The real question is: **What kind of maintenance will you choose for yourself?**

# CHAPTER 10

# YOU ARE NOT YOUR X-RAY

At church three weeks ago, I saw Diane, the 82-year-old who avoided knee replacement and returned to yoga. I usher at our 10:15 a.m. Sunday Mass, and she came up to me and said excitedly, "Dr. P, I'm holding my warrior pose for 30 seconds again. First time in two years. Thank you for giving me my life back."

She hugged me, and I had to sit down for a minute.

Here's a woman who was told she needed surgery, who was told to accept her limitations, who was told that this was just "part of getting older." And now she's talking to me about warrior poses.

That's what this is really about. It's not about x-rays or MRIs or medical procedures. It's about moments of personal victory!

It's about holding a yoga pose and impressing your close friends, that defines who you are instead of watching from the sidelines. It's about walking your dogs through the neighborhood instead of being housebound by pain. It's about maintaining the independence you've fought for your whole life instead of accepting that "this is just how it is now."

It's about waking up in the morning and your first thought being about your day ahead, not about how much your knee hurts.

I know what you might be thinking: *That sounds nice, Dr. P, but my situation is different. My damage is too far along. I've tried everything. I'm too old to start over.*

I've heard those exact words hundreds of times. I've seen the doubt in patients' eyes when they walk into my office feeling defeated by a system that told them they had no choice but to accept pain or undergo surgery.

But here's what I've learned after 30 years of doing this: You are not your x-ray. You are not your MRI. You are not your age or your diagnosis or the number of treatments that haven't worked.

Wayne was told he needed surgery at 43. He avoided it for 23 years.

Randi was told her hiking days were over. She's now planning her family's next dream vacation of a lifetime — this time without the Galapagos nightmares she had prior to getting her knee taken care of.

Bill was convinced he'd never garden or landscape again. He won the neighborhood garden tour last spring.

Jean chose to repair one knee and replace the other just to prove to herself which worked better. The repaired knee won.

And just last month, I got an update from Pam, now 81, who sent me a photo of herself dancing at her grandson's wedding, something she never thought she would be doing the day her knees gave out and she fractured her pelvis.

Every one of them started exactly where you are right now. Skeptical. Tired. Told there was only one option.

You are someone who deserves to feel better. Someone who deserves to move with less pain and more function. Someone who deserves to believe that your best days aren't behind you.

## WHY THIS MATTERS TO ME

Since 1991, I've been working to answer the question I asked as I watched Dr. Murray replace a patient's knee with the very procedure he helped invent: "Is there a way to repair the knee instead of replacing it?"

The Victory Method isn't just a treatment protocol. It's proof that we can help your body heal itself instead of replacing parts with metal, plastic, and cement.

Yes, I love helping my patients repair their joints and regain their movement and quality of life, but what makes this personal for me is when I think about my own granddaughters. One a newborn, and the other not even two years old yet. By the time they're my age — around 2080 — I want them to live in a world where joint replacement surgery is something you read about in history books, not something you fear you might need.

Every patient who avoids surgery, every person who returns to the activities they love, every grandmother like Randi who can play on the beach with her grandchildren — they're all part of something bigger. They're part of my mission to make knee replacements obsolete by 2043.

You could be part of that mission too. Your success doesn't just change your life; it proves to your children and grandchildren that there's a better way forward.

## IMAGINE YOUR FUTURE SELF

Close your eyes for a moment and imagine yourself one year from now. What would it feel like to wake up without that familiar ache in your knee? To stand up from a chair without bracing yourself or thinking about it? To feel stronger and not fear falling? To walk through the grocery store focused on your shopping list instead of calculating how much your joints can handle?

What would it mean to plan a vacation based on where you want to go, not on whether you can physically manage the walking? To accept invitations without first wondering if you'll be able to keep up or having to scout the location to come up with a strategy to make sure the bathrooms are not too far of a walk for you to get to? To offer to help your children or neighbors without worrying about your limitations?

Picture yourself doing something you haven't done in months or years because of your knee pain. Maybe it's dancing at a wedding. Maybe it's hiking a trail you used to love. Maybe it's simply walking through your neighborhood in the evening, enjoying the sunset instead of counting your steps until you can sit down.

Now imagine looking back at this moment — right now, reading this book — as the turning point. The moment you decided you deserved better. The moment you chose hope over resignation.

That future is possible. I see it happen every day in our practice.

## THE PATH FORWARD

You deserve better than the cycle of pills, shots, and doctors telling you to wait until you're ready for surgery. You deserve a doctor who spends more than seven minutes with you. You deserve a plan that treats your whole body, not just your joints.

You deserve hope.

But deserving it and getting it? Those are two different things. Getting it requires taking the first step.

I can't promise you'll be holding a warrior pose at 82 like Diane. I can't guarantee you'll be strolling pain-free on the beach in the Galapagos like Randi or teaching and playing competitive golf like Jerry. Every person is different, and every outcome is unique.

But I can promise you that if you're ready to try something different, if you're ready to invest in yourself and trust a process that's helped 82–95 percent of our patients avoid surgery, then we're ready to help you.

The question isn't whether you can get better. The question is whether you're ready to find out.

## A LEGACY OF HEALING

Think about the people in your life who love you. Your spouse who worries about your pain. Your children who wish they could do something to help. Your grandchildren who don't understand why Grandma or Grandpa can't play certain games anymore.

When you choose to heal — really heal, not just manage symptoms — you're not just changing your own life. You're giving your family back the person they love seeing happy and active. You're modeling for your children the truth that aging doesn't have to mean accepting limitations. You're showing your grandchildren what's possible when you refuse to give up on yourself.

Every success story I've shared with you represents not just one person getting better, but entire families seeing their loved ones flourish; marriages strengthened because partners can enjoy activities together again; grandchildren who get to experience their grandparents as vibrant, active people.

That's the real legacy of choosing repair over replacement, healing over management, hope over resignation.

## YOUR INVITATION

Here's what I want you to consider: What if everything you've been told about your condition is wrong? What if your knee *can* be repaired? What if surgery *isn't* inevitable? What if your body is just waiting for the right support to start healing itself? What if, one year from now, you're the one sending me and my team a text about holding a yoga pose, climbing stairs without pain, or playing with your grandchildren on the beach?

You won't know until you try something different. You won't know until you step outside the system that's been failing you and into an approach that's been succeeding for thousands of people just like you.

As the ancient Chinese proverb states: "The best time to plant a tree was 20 years ago. The second-best time is today."

So...

If the best time to start healing was 20 years ago, the second-best time is *now*!

But first, let me show you exactly what that first step looks like, and how you can take it today.

## CHAPTER 11

# YOUR 21-DAY VICTORY START

You don't have to wait for an appointment to start getting better. In fact, the most powerful healing often begins the moment you decide you're worth fighting for. Over the years, I've learned that patients who prepare their bodies for healing don't just get better results, they reclaim control over their health in a way that transforms everything.

Think about it: you didn't develop your joint problems overnight. Years of inflammation, poor movement patterns, bad mechanics, and systemic stress created the conditions where your body started breaking down faster than it could repair itself. Fortunately, the same body that learned to be in pain can learn to heal.

For decades, I've watched thousands of people discover they had more power over their health than anyone had ever told them. That discovery doesn't start in our office. It starts the moment you decide to stop accepting limitations and start believing your body wants to heal.

That's why the next 21 days are about proving to yourself that change is possible.

# WHY 21 DAYS CHANGES EVERYTHING

"A couple of months prior to seeing you, I was a mess," Mark, a 57-year-old CEO, told me, shaking his head. "My knee and ankle were killing me. The orthopedic surgeon said I needed a knee replacement and even talked about filleting open my Achilles tendon. That scared the hell out of me."

"So, what did you do?" I asked.

"I went online and spent three weeks watching YouTube videos, many of them yours, and researching everything I could about losing weight and reducing inflammation," Mark said. "It was simple stuff I already knew — drink more water, cut sugar and alcohol, eat real food. But once I actually did it, I started sleeping better and had more energy than I'd had in years."

He leaned forward. "Honestly, I almost canceled my appointment with you because I was feeling so much better just from those changes. But thank God I didn't. The MRI showed stress fractures in my knee and a partial Achilles tear — things no amount of water or dieting would have fixed on their own. That's when I realized the prep work wasn't just about feeling better, it was about giving my body a fighting chance once I had the right treatment."

Mark's right. There's a difference between *knowing* what to do and actually *taking action*. Whether you're looking to make a general lifestyle change or you're preparing to begin a joint repair treatment, there's something special about 21 days that goes beyond habit formation. It's long enough for your body to start responding to better choices, but short enough that it doesn't feel overwhelming when you're already dealing with pain.

21 days also gives you proof that you're not broken. You're not too old or too damaged or beyond help. You're someone whose body has been waiting for the right support.

I've seen people reduce their pain levels in the first week just from cutting out inflammatory foods. Others sleep through the night for the first time in months by week two. By week three, most people can feel the difference in their energy levels and how their body moves.

Will 21 days cure your knee or whatever body part is ailing you? Probably not. But it *will* start your body moving in the right direction. And when you do come in for your Clarity Day and Comprehensive Diagnostic Evaluation, your body will be in a much better condition to respond to treatment.

More importantly, you'll know without a doubt that healing is possible.

## YOUR 21-DAY CHALLENGE

If you're ready to take steps toward improving your health, reducing your pain, and increasing your mobility, here's an exact roadmap you can follow for the next 21 days.

> *Always check with your doctor before starting any new diet, exercise, or wellness program.*

### Week 1: Reclaim Your Foundation

The first week isn't about perfection. It's about proving to yourself that small changes can make a real difference. We're going to focus on three areas that have the biggest impact on inflammation and healing.

*1. Increase your daily water intake.*

Chronic dehydration is one of the hidden drivers of joint pain. When you're dehydrated, your joints get stiffer, your inflammation increases, and your body can't transport nutrients where they need to go. Just as importantly, it cannot transport waste and toxins *out* of your body.

Your water goal is simple: Drink half your body weight in ounces every day. So, if you weigh 150 pounds, aim for 75 ounces. If you weigh 200 pounds, aim for 100 ounces.

I know that sounds like a lot if you're not used to drinking water, so I recommend starting with this simple routine:

- 8 ounces first thing when you wake up (before coffee)
- 8 ounces before every meal
- 8 ounces mid-morning and mid-afternoon

That's already 48 ounces, and you haven't even tried yet.

Rick, another one of my patients, admitted, "I've never liked drinking water, and I never realized how much of a difference it could make until I finally started hydrating properly."

He laughed as he recalled, "My girlfriend challenged me to drink one gallon of water a day — that's 128 ounces a day for a month! The loser had to take a cold plunge in Skaneateles Lake, which is very cold in the winter!"

Rick faked a shiver as he continued. "At first, it sounded crazy. I weighed 260 pounds, and when I looked it up online, the general guideline is about half an ounce to an ounce of water per pound of body weight per day. So, I decided to take her up on it. I won, and she had to do the Polar Plunge!"

Aside from the satisfaction of completing the challenge, the physical results he experienced surprised him. "Within three days, I had more energy, I slept better through the night, and my sex life even improved. The trick was drinking most of the water earlier in the day, so I didn't have to get up more than once at night to pee."

## 2. Stop eating inflammatory foods.

Inflammation is like a fire in your body. Every time you eat foods that create inflammation, you're throwing gasoline on that fire. So, for Week 1, you're also going to start removing the gasoline.

*Eliminate the worst inflammatory foods for just one week, including:*

- Fried foods (especially fast food).
- Processed meats (hot dogs, deli meat, cured bacon).
- Foods with ingredients you can't pronounce.

*Cut your sugar intake in half.*

I'm not asking you to eliminate it completely, just cut it in half. If you normally have two sodas a day, have one. If you put two spoonfuls of sugar in your coffee, use one. If you eat dessert every night, make it every other night.

*Add one anti-inflammatory food per day, such as:*

- A handful of berries.
- A serving of leafy greens.
- Fatty fish (salmon, sardines, mackerel).
- A handful of nuts (especially walnuts).
- A cup of green tea.

Don't overthink this. Just pick one and stick with it for the week.

*3. Acknowledge where you are so you can see where you're going.*

This might be the most important part of week one, and it's the part most people want to skip. Keep a simple pain journal. Every evening, write down three things:

1. What did my pain stop me from doing today?
2. How did I feel about that?
3. What's one thing I want to be able to do again?

Don't make this complicated. Just write a few sentences. The goal isn't to dwell on your problems; it's to get clear about what you're working with.

When I first introduced the idea of keeping a simple pain journal to Susan, she wrinkled her nose. "I don't want to sit around writing about everything that's wrong with me," she said.

"It's not about problems," I explained. "It's about clarity. If you don't acknowledge what's limiting you, you can't measure your progress."

Reluctantly, she agreed. A week later, she came back, journal in hand. "I had no idea how much I was holding myself back," she admitted. "I wrote that my pain stopped me from playing with my grandkids, and then I realized that I wasn't even trying anymore. That broke my heart."

She looked at me with tears in her eyes and said, "Now I know what I want: I want to be able to get down on the floor with them again. Writing it down made me see that's my real goal. And for the first time in years, I believe it's possible."

That awareness is the first step toward change. You can't heal what you don't acknowledge.

## Week 2: Movement is Medicine

Now that you've started building your foundation, we're going to add gentle movement and targeted support. Your body was designed to move, and movement is medicine — but it has to be the right kind of movement. For week two, we're focusing on safe, beneficial movement that reminds your body how good it feels to move without pain.

### 1. Begin taking daily walks.

Start with 10-15 minutes every day. If that's too much, start with five minutes. If you can already walk for 30 minutes, don't increase it yet — we're building consistency, not intensity. Walk on flat surfaces if possible. If the weather's bad, walk inside at the gym, a mall, your hallway, or wherever you can move safely.

## 2. Implement a gentle range of motion routine.

Twice a day, spend five minutes moving your knee (or whatever body part is bothering you) through its full range of motion. Here is a simple routine you can follow:

- Sitting in a chair, straighten your leg as much as comfortable, then bend it as much as comfortable
- Do this slowly, 10–15 times

If this motion hurts, back off. This should feel like a gentle stretch, not pain.

## 3. Listen to your body.

If something makes your pain worse, don't do it. The goal is consistent, gentle movement, not heroic efforts that set you back. Movement is medicine.

Pair these new routines with your Week 1 habits. Keep up with your water intake, dietary changes, and pain journaling. By now, some of these should be starting to feel more automatic.

## Week 3: Integration and Preparation

The final week is about bringing everything together and preparing for your next steps. By now, you should have a good sense of what's working for you and what isn't.

## 1. Refine your routine.

Double down on the changes that are making you feel better. Maybe you've discovered that cutting sugar made a bigger difference than you expected. Maybe walking after dinner helps you sleep better. Maybe drinking more water has improved your energy.

Pay attention to these patterns; *this is where journaling helps the most.* Your body is telling you what it needs.

## 2. *Optimize your sleep.*

Poor sleep makes everything worse — pain, inflammation, heal-ing, and mood. For week three, focus on improving your sleep quality, because that's when your body does most of its healing.

Create a wind-down routine and start preparing for sleep an hour before bedtime. You can do that by following these simple steps:

- Dim the lights.
- Put away screens (phones, tablets, TV).
- Try some gentle stretching or deep breathing.
- Consider a warm bath with Epsom salts.

If you're still having trouble sleeping, consider these natural options, but always confirm with your own doctor and pharmacist:

- Melatonin (start with 0.5-1mg, taken 30 minutes before bed)
- Magnesium glycinate (200-400mg taken 30 minutes before bed)
- Chamomile tea

Remember, good sleep is when your body does most of its healing. Prioritize it.

## Prepare for Your Next Step

By the end of 21 days, you should have a clearer picture of your condition and what's working for you. Use this information to decide on your next step. Ask yourself the following questions:

- How much improvement have I seen in 21 days?
- What changes made the biggest difference?
- What areas still need professional attention?
- Am I ready to invest in a comprehensive approach?

# WHAT TO EXPECT
# (AND WHY SMALL CHANGES MATTER)

Everyone sees different results in 21 days, but here's what I typically hear:

- **Week 1:** "I'm sleeping better and have more energy."
- **Week 2:** "My pain isn't gone, but it's not as constant."
- **Week 3:** "I can do things I couldn't do three weeks ago."

Some people see dramatic improvements. Others see subtle changes. Both are normal and valuable. The important thing isn't how much you improve in 21 days; it's that you start moving in the right direction. You're proving to yourself that your body responds to better choices. You're building confidence that healing is possible.

Remember, you didn't develop your knee problem in 21 days, and you probably won't solve it completely in 21 days either. But you can definitely start the healing process.

## Proof that Prep Work Pays Off

"I'd been pushing through shoulder pain for years," Carl told me. "Lifting, working out, doing whatever I had to do — no matter what, I was always dealing with the pain."

When I asked him why he finally committed to the 21-day prep, he said, "I realized the healthier I was going in, the better the outcome. So, I cut out alcohol, tightened up my diet, stuck with organic meats, and got serious about my stretching and exercises."

"The hardest part?" he admitted with a grin. "Holding myself back from heavy lifting. I'm wired to just suck it up and do what's needed, but this time I had to train differently."

Four weeks after his procedure, Carl looked at me and shook his head. "My shoulder is moving better than it has since my surgery three years ago. And honestly? Cutting alcohol gave me more energy, mental clarity, even a better mood.

The prep didn't just set me up for healing, it changed the way I feel about my health."

# BEYOND 21 DAYS: YOUR NEXT STEPS

After three weeks of preparing your body for healing, you'll be ready to take the next step in your journey. If you're seeing good improvements and want to continue on your own, keep doing what's working. Add in more anti-inflammatory foods, increase your walking gradually, and consider working with a nutritionist or personal trainer who understands joint health.

If you're seeing some improvement but know you need more comprehensive help, that's where a Clarity Day comes in. Like I described in Chapter 6, your Clarity Day is when we can complete a comprehensive assessment to discover exactly what's happening in your body and what's possible for your healing.

## Smart Questions to Ask Any Provider

Whether you decide to work with us or explore other options, here are some questions you should ask any healthcare provider:

- How much time will you spend with me at each visit?
- What's your success rate with patients like me?
- Do you address the whole body or just the joint and painful body parts?
- What happens if the first treatment doesn't work?
- How do you track and measure progress?
- What's your philosophy on surgery, when do you feel it's necessary, and when can it be avoided?
- Do you have any kind of guarantee?

These questions will help you find a provider who truly understands comprehensive healing, not just symptom management. Visit the References section at the back of the book to access a more comprehensive list of questions you can ask your provider.

## YOUR TIME IS NOW

You have a choice to make. You can continue down the path you've been on — managing symptoms, hoping for the best, accepting that pain is just part of getting older.

Or you can try something different.

You can invest in yourself. You can believe that your body has the ability to heal. You can take the first step toward the life you want to be living.

I won't tell you it's easy. Nothing worth doing is easy. But I will tell you it is definitely possible. I've seen it happen thousands of times, including for me! Start with your 21 days. See what's possible when you start giving your body what it needs to heal itself.

Your journey toward a pain-free life can start today. The only question is: *Are you ready to take the first step?*

All you have to do is decide that you deserve better — because you do.

Start working to repair your joints and join the movement to make the world #KneeReplacementFreeBy43.

# ENDING THE NEED FOR KNEE REPLACEMENTS BY 2043

Before laying out this roadmap, it is worth remembering President John F. Kennedy's challenge to America in the early 1960s. In an address to Congress and again at Rice University, he declared that we would put a man on the moon and return him safely to Earth before the decade was over. At the time, our technological limitations made this sound impossible, yet in 1969, it was accomplished. If we could achieve that with mid-20th-century tools, then surely by 2043, with current and emerging technology, we can end the need for knee replacements.

So, using Ed Rush's *God Talks* techniques, I decided to sit down in a dark, quiet, peaceful location, close my eyes, and ask God the lies and truths about #KneeReplacementFreeBy43. What follows is what He revealed to me.

On January 1, 2043, I will stand in a museum of medical history and point to a stainless-steel (actually cobalt-chrome, but stay with me here) knee. Children will stare at it the way we stare at leeches and bone saws — curious, a little horrified, and grateful we've moved on.

This roadmap for ending knee replacements is how we can get there.

I am building a movement that replaces resignation with repair. For decades, people have been told there are only two choices:

1. Tough it out — or worse yet, "suck it up."
2. Get it replaced.

That ends with this book. We are scaling the third option — Knee Repair, NOT Knee Replacement — from one clinic to a worldwide standard.

## PHASE 1: PROOF AT SCALE (NOW → 2028)

I will turn our daily work into undeniable evidence. Not slogans, but data sets. We already have the DataBiologics national registry I wrote about earlier in the book. We will continue partnering with them and other clinics to share information, collaborate, refine methods, and accelerate results to create *synergy*! Together, we will track outcomes, function returned, pain lessened, and lives reclaimed so that we can all get better at repairing knees and other joints rather than replacing them.

Within three years, we will have three Victory In Motion clinics, home of the Knee Repair, NOT Knee Replacement approach, and eight to 10 affiliate partnership sites in diverse health systems in private, academic, rural, and urban settings. Each will operate under the same repair-first clinical pathways and training, aligned with our model, and all will report to the DataBiologics registry. These partnerships will expand our reach while maintaining consistency and quality, ensuring every site reflects the same philosophy and results.

We will also attack the problem from the front end by cutting tomorrow's surgeries through prevention. We will partner with middle schools, high schools, colleges, and youth club sports to implement Sportsmetrics-style neuromuscular training and injury-prevention programs. The data is clear: Targeted programs can slash serious knee injuries, especially ACL tears. Females suffer ACL tears at far higher rates than males, but both groups benefit when prevention programs are adopted. And when ACL tears drop, future osteoarthritis drops with them, and then — you guessed it — if arthritis drops, the need for joint replacements drops.

Prevention goes beyond sports. By implementing weight management and anti-inflammatory lifestyle programs early in school settings — like those started by celebrity chef Jamie Oliver and Prime Minister Tony Blair in England — we will further reduce the risk and progression of arthritis across all ages. **We are what we eat**, and nutrition, especially genetic-based nutrition counseling, is a must.

We will also continue to advance the frontier of ACL repair. The Bridge-Enhanced ACL Restoration (BEAR®) surgery — the #SaveTheACL movement — is showing great promise. In animal studies, BEAR repairs did not develop arthritis, while standard ACL reconstructions and untreated ACL tears did. Early human trial data are trending the same way, and within the next several years we should know definitively if BEAR repairs cut the risk of arthritis in humans. If confirmed, this will be a landmark moment in orthopedic surgery.

And we won't stop there. We will push ACL repair to the next level by combining BEAR with biologics such as bone marrow aspirate cells and PRP, just as we are already doing in practice. Repairing, rather than replacing or reconstructing, is the future, and BEAR is proof that repair-first thinking saves joints today and can potentially prevent arthritis tomorrow.

We will continue to push the boundaries of ACL, other knee ligaments, meniscus cartilage and articular cartilage repair, and non-operative treatments expanding and helping improve non-operative techniques such as Cross Bracing Protocol (CBP) and regenerative medicine repair techniques with biologic treatments.

We will not stop until we have a true "Dr. Bones McCoy Star Trek tricorder" device to both diagnose and treat injuries and illnesses completely noninvasively and nonoperatively. I've had that dream since my childhood watching Star Trek — that day will come, my friends!

## PHASE 2: EARLY DETECTION BECOMES ROUTINE (2027 → 2030)

This phase focuses on prevention and proactive action. We will develop screening systems and protocols to identify at-risk patients earlier than ever before. This includes genetic testing and screening plus the routine use of x-rays and specialized MRI scans not just to look at cartilage, but to detect the earliest signs of subchondral stress/microfracturing. These bone changes are far easier to repair if caught early, and the earlier they are addressed, repaired, and heal, the lower the lifetime risk of developing arthritis.

Compositional MRIs that reveal cartilage matrix changes before morphology collapses will become more common, giving us a window into damage at its earliest stage. At the same time, we will work to develop new diagnostic technologies not yet available today, knowing that the breakthroughs of tomorrow will be essential to making this roadmap real. It is awe-inspiring to even start to think about all of the unknown or as yet undeveloped tools, techniques, treatments, and programs that will be discovered and developed over the next five to 10 years that will be the golden age of regenerative medicine!

Biomarkers will also become routine. We will analyze blood, urine, and synovial fluid for increasingly well-defined molecular markers that reveal cartilage breakdown, inflammation, and joint health years before arthritis becomes visible on traditional imaging.

Wearables and smartphone-based gait and load analysis will give us real-time data about how knees and other joints are stressed in everyday life. Combined with artificial intelligence, we will integrate all of this data — imaging, biomarkers, biomechanics, and risk factors — into precision screening, prevention, and treatment programs tailored for each individual.

Throughout this phase, we will continue to push for new technology, including tools still in early development or not even conceived of yet, because that is what it will take to transform care from reactive to preventive.

## PHASE 3: THE MOONSHOT TRIALS (2030 → 2035)

This is our moonshot. We will coordinate with the leading societies and organizations in cartilage repair, arthritis research, regenerative medicine, and orthopedics to launch large, adaptive, multi-center trials that put repair, prevention, and regeneration head-to-head against the status quo.

These trials will not test one injection versus another. They will test entire systems of care — advanced diagnostics; cell-based therapies; PRP; a broad range of biologics, including exosomes, extracellular vesicles, and cytokines; emerging and yet-to-be-discovered signaling molecules; biomechanics and gait retraining; metabolic and weight-loss programs; anti-inflammatory nutrition; bioidentical hormone therapy; functional medicine; and overall wellness.

Every arm will be integrated, comprehensive, and future-focused. We will measure not just pain relief, but joint survival without replacement, restoration of function, cost savings, and quality of life.

Artificial intelligence will be the engine that ties it all together. AI will integrate data across sites, harmonize protocols, and identify best practices faster than human analysis alone. It will learn from imaging, biomarkers, outcomes, and lifestyle inputs to recommend and refine treatment plans in real time.

These Moonshot Trials will provide the undeniable evidence needed to shift global practice: showing that a comprehensive, repair-first, proactive, prevention-focused pathway outperforms the outdated surgery-first mindset.

## PHASE 4: CHANGE THE INCENTIVES (2030 →2036)

We cannot change medicine without changing the incentives. Right now, the system rewards surgery volume. That has to end. During this phase, we will design and implement value-based payment models that reward keeping people out of the operating room. Bundled payments, shared-savings contracts, and outcome-based reimbursements will make prevention, early detection, and durable repair financially sustainable for health systems and attractive for providers.

The Centers for Medicare and Medicaid Services and private insurers already define function, cost, and complications as the endpoints they care about. We will meet those endpoints with real-world data from our registry and Moonshot Trials, proving that a repair-first pathway delivers superior outcomes at lower cost. By aligning payment with preservation instead of replacement, we will flip the economic engine of orthopedics from reactive surgery to proactive repair.

## PHASE 5: NORMALIZE REPAIR, RETIRE REPLACEMENT (2035 → 2043)

By the mid-2030s, repair will no longer be the exception, it will be the default. With confirmatory trial data, trained centers, payer alignment, and widespread cultural adoption, repair-first and prevention-first care will be the standard, while replacement becomes the rare fallback.

National registries will add a "Replacements Avoided" metric alongside procedure counts, and year by year, that number will climb. By 2040, the curve of knee replacements will be bending down sharply, and the cobalt-chrome and titanium knee will be headed for the medical museum.

## THE ENGINES THAT POWER THE ROADMAP

### 1. The $1 vs. $1M Challenge – The War Chest

At least $1 from every book sale and every donation fuels this mission, whether it comes from a student or a philanthropist. The funnel makes it simple: donate, gift a book, become an ambassador. Millions of small contributions add up to the movement that ends replacements. When the last knee replacement is performed and knee replacements (and eventually all artificial joint replacements) are no longer needed, this book is no longer needed because it will be obsolete and will be retired.

### 2. The Victory Academy – Training a Repair-First Workforce

We will build a training and certification system for providers via Victory In Motion centers and affiliate sites to replicate the model.

Within a decade, thousands of clinicians will be trained in repair-first clinical pathways, so the philosophy and results spread far beyond our walls.

### 3. The Open Registry – Radical Transparency

We will continue partnering with DataBiologics and other open registries to publish real-world outcomes. Every knee saved from replacement becomes part of the data. Transparent, independent reporting will drive credibility, accountability, and constant improvement.

## 4. The Prevention Ladder – Cutting Off the Problem at the Root

We will hard-wire prevention into schools, sports programs, and communities to reduce ACL tears and other joint injuries. Females remain at higher risk than males, but both benefit when prevention is routine.

Prevention also includes promoting lifestyle changes. For every pound of body weight lost, three to four pounds of force are taken off the knee joint.[26] Combine this with anti-inflammatory nutrition, total-body fitness, and exercise, and the arthritis and knee replacement curves begin to flatten before they even start.

## 5. The Early-OA Checkup – New Vital Signs

Every annual checkup will include a Joint Health Panel that includes imaging, biomarkers, gait analysis, and AI-driven risk scoring. This shifts detection from late-stage to early-stage and makes proactive repair the norm.

## 6. The Surgical Pivot – Industry as Ally

Joint replacement manufacturers must pivot from metal and plastic to biologics, 3D printing, better tissue engineering, and regenerative solutions. They must come to understand that they are not in the implant business; they are in the mobility business. We will partner with them to accelerate the shift.

## 7. The Story Engine – Culture Change

Data alone is not enough. We will tell stories of grandparents walking stairs again, athletes spared from ACL tears, and retirees hiking pain-free — and we will pair those stories with hard numbers. Stories move hearts; data moves systems. Together, they create the culture shift that retires replacement.

## THE PLEDGE

I will measure our success by replacements avoided, pain relieved, function restored, lives unshackled, and goals and dreams achieved. I will develop and make available the playbook, publish the numbers, and invite critique. I will keep preventive, proactive, functional, and regenerative medicine first, and I will continue refining the program as new science arrives, leveraging the power of AI to accelerate every step.

And when we place that last knee implant in the museum, I will smile, close the book that helped get us there, and be grateful it is finally obsolete.

Knee Repair, NOT Knee Replacement.

#KneeReplacementFreeBy43

## JOIN THE MOVEMENT

If what you've just read excites you — if you believe, deep down, that the world can and should move beyond metal, plastic, and cement replacements — then you belong with us.

Victory In Motion, home of Knee Repair, NOT Knee Replacement, is always looking for talented, passionate individuals who want to be part of this mission. Whether your background is in medicine, fitness, wellness, technology, administration, or simply helping people live without limits, we want to meet you.

If you're ready to join the movement, scan the QR code below or visit www.VictoryInMotion.com. You can also reach us at 1-315-993-KNEE to learn more about current opportunities.

Together, let's change the future of musculoskeletal health and make the world #KneeReplacementFreeBy43!

Join The Movement

# ENDNOTES

1    American College of Rheumatology. "Total Knee and Hip Replacement Surgeries Are Modern-Day Miracles." *AnMed Orthopedics & Sports Medicine*, November 9, 2023. https://anmed.org/wellness/blog/total-knee-and-hip-replacement-surgeries-help-millions

2    Vanessa Lam, Steven Teutsch, and Jonathan Fielding, "Hip and Knee Replacements: A Neglected Potential Savings Opportunity," *JAMA* 319, no. 10 (March 13, 2018): 977–78, https://doi.org/10.1001/jama.2018.2310; Dowsey, Michelle M., Jane Gunn, and Peter F. M. Choong. "Selecting Those to Refer for Joint Replacement: Who Will Likely Benefit and Who Will Not?" *Best Practice & Research Clinical Rheumatology* 28, no. 1 (2014): 157–71. https://doi.org/10.1016/j.berh.2014.01.005.

3    Gunaratne, Raveendhara R., Dylan J. Pratt, Mark B. Banda, David F. Fick, and R. Mark Gollish. "Patient Dissatisfaction Following Total Knee Arthroplasty: A Systematic Review." *The Journal of Arthroplasty* 32, no. 12 (2017): 3854–60. https://doi.org/10.1016/j.arth.2017.07.021; Wylde, Vikki, Andrew Beswick, Jonathan Bruce, Ashley Blom, Nigel Howells, and Rachael Gooberman-Hill. "Chronic Pain after Total Knee Arthroplasty." *EFORT Open Reviews* 3, no. 8 (2018): 461–70. https://doi.org/10.1302/2058-5241.3.180004 (Free full text: https://pmc.ncbi.nlm.nih.gov/articles/PMC6134884/)

4    Riddle, D. L., Macfarlane, G. J., Hamilton, D. F., Beasley, M., & Dumenci, L. (2022). "Cross-validation of good

versus poor self-reported outcome trajectory types following knee arthroplasty." *Osteoarthritis and Cartilage*, 30(1), 61–68. https://doi.org/10.1016/j.joca.2021.09.004

5   DataBiologics is a national outcomes registry that tracks real-world data from regenerative medicine clinics across the US to measure patient-reported outcomes, pain reduction, function restoration, and satisfaction rates in a standardized way.

6   Renub Research, "Knee Replacement Market Size, Competitors & Forecast to 2032," *Research and Markets*, October 2024. Accessed October 2024, https://www.researchandmarkets.com/report/knee-replacement?srsltid=AfmBOoob8carY27ziUEXHit-GSpIXRQNMjqG4FRttV9F4aRZDpr2fZIC.

7   McAlindon, Timothy E., Michael J. LaValley, William F. Harvey, Jeffrey B. Driban, Ming Zhang, Lori Lyn Price, Robert J. Ward. 2017. "Effect of Intra-articular Triamcinolone vs Saline on Knee Cartilage Volume and Pain in Patients With Knee Osteoarthritis: A Randomized Clinical Trial." *JAMA* 317 (19): 1967–75. https://doi.org/10.1001/jama.2017.5283; Wernecke, C., S. E. Braun, and K. M. Dragoo. "Intra-Articular Corticosteroid Injections: A Systematic Review of Their Effects on Articular Cartilage." *Orthopaedic Journal of Sports Medicine* 3, no. 5 (2015): 2325967115581163; https://doi.org/10.1177/2325967115581163; Therapeutic Trajectory Following Intra-Articular Hyaluronic Acid Injection in Knee Osteoarthritis: A Meta-Analysis." *Osteoarthritis and Cartilage* 19, no. 6 (2011): 611–619. https://doi.org/10.1016/j.joca.2010.09.014.

8   Hewett, Timothy E., and Nathaniel A. Bates. "Preventive Biomechanics: A Paradigm Shift with a Translational Approach to Injury Prevention." *American Journal of Sports Medicine* 45, no. 1 (2017): 261–270. https://doi.org/10.1177/0363546516686080; Myer, Gregory D., Kevin R. Ford, and Timothy E. Hewett. "Methodological Approaches and Rationale for Training to Prevent Anterior Cruciate Ligament Injuries in Female Athletes." *Scandinavian*

*Journal of Medicine & Science in Sports* 17, no. 3 (2007): 252–265. https://doi.org/10.1111/j.1600-0838.2004.00410.x.

9   According to DataBiologics, a national outcomes registry that tracks real-world data from regenerative medicine clinics across the US to measure patient-reported outcomes, pain reduction, function restoration, and satisfaction rates in a standardized way.

10  Bharadwaj, U. U., Link, T. M., Akkaya, Z., Joseph, G. B., Kumar, D., Souza, R. B., Baum, T., Lane, N. E., Nevitt, M. C., Lynch, J. A., & Li, X. "Intra-Articular Knee Injections and Progression of Knee Osteoarthritis: Data from the Osteoarthritis Initiative." *Radiological Society of North America*, May 27, 2025. https://pubs.rsna.org/doi/10.1148/radiol.233081; Darbandi, A., Hormozian, S., Pooyan, A., Demehri, S., & Guermazi, A. (2022, November 29). Medial joint space narrowing and Kellgren-Lawrence progression following intra-articular corticosteroid injections compared to hyaluronic acid injections and nontreated patients. In Radiological Society of North America (RSNA) Annual Meeting, Chicago, IL.

11  Wang, et al. "The Optimal Time To Inject Bone Mesenchymal Stem Cells For Fracture Healing In A Murine Model." *Stem Cell Research & Therapy*, 2018. https://stemcellres.biomedcentral.com/articles/10.1186/s13287-018-1034-7; Laidding, S. R., et al. "Effect of Bone Marrow Aspirate Concentrate–Platelet-Rich Plasma on Tendon-Derived Stem Cells and Rotator Cuff Tendon Tear." *Journal of Orthopaedic Research*, 2017. https://www.researchgate.net/publication/312587504_Effect_of_Bone_Marrow_Aspirate_Concentrate_Platelet-Rich_Plasma_on_Tendon_Derived_Stem_Cells_and_Rotator_Cuff_Tendon_Tear; Themistocleous, G. S., et al. "Effectiveness of a Single Intra-Articular Bone Marrow Aspirate Concentrate Injection in Patients with Grade 3 and 4 Knee Osteoarthritis." World Journal of Orthopaedics 9, no. 7 (2018): 112–18. https://pmc.ncbi.nlm.nih.gov/articles/PMC6197942/

12  Stenderup, K., J. Justesen, E. F. Eriksen, S. I. S. Rattan, and M. Kassem. "Number and Proliferative Capacity of Osteogenic Stem Cells Are Maintained during Aging and in Patients with Osteoporosis." *Journal of Bone and Mineral Research* 16, no. 6 (2001): 1120–29. https://doi.org/10.1359/jbmr.2001.16.6.1120; Hernigou, Philippe, Jérôme Delambre, Steffen Quiennec, and Alexandre Poignard. "Human Bone Marrow Mesenchymal Stem Cell Injection in Subchondral Lesions of Knee Osteoarthritis: A Prospective Randomized Study versus Contralateral Arthroplasty at a Mean Fifteen Year Follow-Up." *International Orthopaedics* 45 (2021): 365–73. https://doi.org/10.1007/s00264-020-04571-4

13  Cobos, Raquel, Amaia Latorre, Felipe Aizpuru, Juan I. Guenaga, Clara Sarasqueta, Antonio Escobar, Jaime L. Fernández-Sainz, et al. 2010. "Variability of Indication Criteria in Knee and Hip Replacement: An Observational Study." *BMC Musculoskeletal Disorders* 11 (1): 249. https://doi.org/10.1186/1471-2474-11-249; Riddle, Daniel L., William A. Jiranek, and Curtis W. Hayes. 2014. "Use of a Validated Algorithm to Judge the Appropriateness of Total Knee Arthroplasty in the United States: A Multicenter Longitudinal Cohort Study." *Arthritis & Rheumatology* 66 (8): 2134–43. https://doi.org/10.1002/art.38685

14  Eppley, Barry L., Jeffrey E. Woodell, and James Higgins. "Platelet Quantification and Growth Factor Analysis from Platelet-Rich Plasma: Implications for Wound Healing." *Plastic and Reconstructive Surgery* 114, no. 6 (2004): 1502–1508. https://doi.org/10.1097/01.PRS.0000138251.07040.51; Kawase, Takanori, Kenji Okuda, Larry F. Wolff, and Hiroshi Yoshie. "Platelet-Rich Plasma-Derived Fibrin Clot Formation Stimulates Release of Growth Factors and Cytokines from Platelets and Leukocytes." *Journal of Periodontology* 74, no. 6 (2003): 849–857. https://doi.org/10.1902/jop.2003.74.6.849

15  Scher, C., Craig, J. & Nelson, F. Bone marrow edema in the knee in osteoarthrosis and association with total

knee arthroplasty within a three-year follow-up. *Skeletal Radiology*. 37, 609–617 (2008). https://doi.org/10.1007/s00256-008-0504-x

16  Li, Weiqiang, Qianqian Liu, Jinchao Shi, Xiang Xu, and Jinyi Xu. "The Role of TNF-α in the Fate Regulation and Functional Reprogramming of Mesenchymal Stem Cells in an Inflammatory Microenvironment." *Frontiers in Immunology* 14 (February 6, 2023). https://doi.org/10.3389/fimmu.2023.1074863; Wehling, N., G. D. Palmer, C. Pilapil, F. Liu, J. W. Wells, P. E. Müller, C. H. Evans, and R. M. Porter. "Interleukin-1βκ and Tumor Necrosis Factor α Inhibit Chondrogenesis by Human Mesenchymal Stem Cells through NF-κB–Dependent Pathways." *Arthritis & Rheumatism* 60, no. 3 (February 26, 2009): 801–12. https://doi.org/10.1002/art.24352; Ho, Nicole Pui-Yu, and Hitoshi Takizawa. "Inflammation Regulates Haematopoietic Stem Cells and Their Niche." *International Journal of Molecular Sciences* 23, no. 3 (January 20, 2022): 1125. https://doi.org/10.3390/ijms23031125

17  Kilroe, Sean P., Jonathan Fulford, Sarah R. Jackman, Luc J. Van Loon, and Benjamin T. Wall. "Temporal Muscle-Specific Disuse Atrophy during One Week of Leg Immobilization." *Medicine & Science in Sports & Exercise* 52, no. 4 (November 4, 2019): 944–54. https://doi.org/10.1249/mss.0000000000002200; Hardy, Edward J., Thomas B. Inns, Jacob Hatt, Brett Doleman, Joseph J. Bass, Philip J. Atherton, Jonathan N. Lund, and Bethan E. Phillips. "The Time Course of Disuse Muscle Atrophy of the Lower Limb in Health and Disease." *Journal of Cachexia, Sarcopenia and Muscle* 13, no. 6 (September 14, 2022): 2616–29. https://doi.org/10.1002/jcsm.13067.

18  Di Martino, Alessandro, Berardo Di Matteo, Tiziana Papio, Francesco Tentoni, Filippo Selleri, Annarita Cenacchi, Elizaveta Kon, and Giuseppe Filardo. "Platelet-Rich Plasma versus Hyaluronic Acid Injections for the Treatment of Knee Osteoarthritis: Results at 5 Years of a Double-Blind, Randomized Controlled Trial." *The American Journal of*

*Sports Medicine* 47, no. 2 (December 13, 2018): 347–54. https://doi.org/10.1177/0363546518814532; Hernigou, P., Auregan, J.C., Dubory, A. et al. "Subchondral stem cell therapy versus contralateral total knee arthroplasty for osteoarthritis following secondary osteonecrosis of the knee." *International Orthopaedics* (SICOT) 42, 2563–2571 (2018). https://doi.org/10.1007/s00264-018-3916-9

19 Exercise for Osteoarthritis of the Knee." Cochrane Database of Systematic Reviews 2015, no. 1 (CD004376). https://doi.org/10.1002/14651858.CD004376.pub3; Messier, Stephen P., Shannon L. Mihalko, Claudine Legault, et al. "Effects of Intensive Diet and Exercise on Knee Joint Loads, Inflammation, and Clinical Outcomes among Overweight and Obese Adults with Knee Osteoarthritis." *JAMA* 310, no. 12 (September 25, 2013): 1263. https://doi.org/10.1001/jama.2013.277669

20 Prasanna, Shreya S., Nicol Korner-Bitensky, and Sara Ahmed. "Why Do People Delay Accessing Health Care for Knee Osteoarthritis? Exploring Beliefs of Health Professionals and Lay People." *Physiotherapy Canada* 65, no. 1 (January 2013): 56–63. https://doi.org/10.3138/ptc.2011-50; Velek, P., E. de Schepper, D. Schiphof, et al. "Changes to Consultations and Diagnosis of Osteoarthritis in Primary Care during the COVID-19 Pandemic." *Osteoarthritis and Cartilage* 31, no. 6 (June 2023): 829–38. https://doi.org/10.1016/j.joca.2023.02.075

21 Scher, C., Craig, J. & Nelson, F. Bone marrow edema in the knee in osteoarthrosis and association with total knee arthroplasty within a three-year follow-up. *Skeletal Radiology.* 37, 609–617 (2008). https://doi.org/10.1007/s00256-008-0504-x

22 MoneyGeek. "Average Price of a New Car in 2025." November 2025. https://www.moneygeek.com/resources/average-price-of-a-new-car/; Experian. *Automotive Consumer Insight Report.* May 2025. https://www.experian.com/blogs/ask-experian/average-car-price/

23 Volpi, Elena, Reza Nazemi, and Satoshi Fujita. "Muscle Tissue Changes with Aging." *Current Opinion in Clinical Nutrition and Metabolic Care* 7, no. 4 (July 2004): 405–10. https://doi.org/10.1097/01.mco.0000134362.76653.b2

24 Watson, Steven L, Benjamin K Weeks, Lisa J Weis, Amy T Harding, Sean A Horan, and Belinda R Beck. "High-Intensity Resistance and Impact Training Improves Bone Mineral Density and Physical Function in Postmenopausal Women with Osteopenia and Osteoporosis: The LIFTMOR Randomized Controlled Trial." *Journal of Bone and Mineral Research* 33, no. 2 (October 4, 2017): 211–20. https://doi.org/10.1002/jbmr.3284.

25 Westcott, Wayne L. "Resistance Training Is Medicine." *Current Sports Medicine Reports* 11, no. 4 (2012): 209–16. https://doi.org/10.1249/jsr.0b013e31825dabb8

26 Messier SP, Gutekunst DJ, Davis C, DeVita P., "Weight loss reduces knee-joint loads in overweight and obese older adults with knee osteoarthritis," *Arthritis & Rheumatism*, 2005 Jul;52(7):2026-2032. DOI:10.1002/art.21139. URL: https://pubmed.ncbi.nlm.nih.gov/15986358/

# THIS BOOK INCLUDES
# FREE RESOURCES
## TO HELP YOU BEGIN YOUR HEALING JOURNEY TODAY

### USE THE QR CODE BELOW TO CLAIM YOURS.

#### "Can This Help Me?" Self-Assessment

A simple quiz to help you understand if you're
a good candidate for The Victory Method.

#### Smart Questions to Ask Any Provider

Your guide to getting the answers you deserve.

#### 21-Day Victory Start Email Series

Daily tips and encouragement sent right to your inbox.

Free Resources

## VictoryInMotion.com/RepairNotReplaceBook

# HOW THIS BOOK CAME TO BE

The February night air was cool, but this was Las Vegas, and the winter temperatures were nowhere near as biting as what I was used to in Upstate New York. Funnel Hacking Live 2025, Russell Brunson's annual high-energy business conference for entrepreneurs, had just begun, and I was currently standing inside Blake Shelton's Ole Red bar at an invite-only, pre-conference party.

The place was jam-packed with hundreds of entrepreneurs. Loud country music and the smell of barbecue filled the air. After weaving through the crowd to order a Newcastle Brown Ale at the bar, I finally found a seat overlooking the stage. A few moments later, Russell Brunson walked out, and the energy in the room shifted from casual networking to something more akin to a rock concert.

Two women sat down next to me.

"Hi, I'm Christina."

"Hi, I'm Nicole."

Before I could ask them what they did for a living, they beat me to it. Christina was a singer/songwriter, and Nicole said she was a book publisher. I shared my elevator speech in return. "Hi, I'm Dr. Marc Pietropaoli, Founder and CEO of Victory In Motion, home of Knee Repair, NOT Knee Replacement — a program that helps people avoid having their knees and other body parts replaced by using their own body's natural ability to heal itself."

Christina perked right up. "My ankle is a mess. It hurts every day." I gave her ankle a quick look and offered some advice about what exercises to do and what to avoid.

Nicole asked me if I'd ever thought about writing a book, and I laughed and admitted that everyone had been telling me to write a book for years, but I was terrified. I had no idea how to start, what to do, or even if I could pull it off. I told her I was working with Vince Green, a business coach, and that he'd promised to connect me with a publisher.

What I didn't know was that the woman sitting right next to me in this loud, crowded bar — Nicole Gebhardt, owner of Niche Press — was the very publisher Vince had in mind.

Once we'd figured out that Nicole was the person Vince wanted to recommend, the realization hit me like a ton of bricks. Out of the hundreds of people currently standing in this four-story bar in Las Vegas, the person who had been recommended to help me write my first book just *happened* to sit next to me! I knew in that instant meeting Nicole wasn't a coincidence — it was God's plan.

Nicole and I connected deeply over the next few days and eventually agreed to work together. From then on, I pursued the calling to finally write the book that had been in me for years.

She introduced me to her amazing team at Niche Press and soon sent me a welcome package with two books inside: *Storytelling Made Easy* by Michael Hauge, the man who'd trained Russell Brunson and Hollywood stars like Will Smith on the art of storytelling and his approach to the hero's two journeys, and *God Talks* by Ed Rush, a retired Marine fighter pilot.

Interestingly, the three things I wanted to be when I was growing up were a rockstar drummer like Keith Moon of The Who, a Marine fighter pilot like those in the show *Black Sheep Squadron*, or a sports medicine doctor. I had to "settle" for becoming a sports medicine doctor since my eyes were not good enough to be a fighter pilot at the time, and my parents would have killed me if I'd skipped college to become a rock and roll drummer.

*This was meant to be,* I thought as I skimmed the front and back covers of Ed's book.

I devoured both books. Michael taught me how to shape my stories into something emotionally powerful. Ed taught me how to stop simply talking to God and start listening. That practice alone began transforming my life and my business.

But the path to publication wasn't easy. Writing this book meant wrestling with many long days and nights, old fears, and constant doubts. I kept asking myself, *What if nobody cares? What if the book isn't good enough?*

Some of these fears and false beliefs stemmed from my past when I carried the weight of being a busy orthopedic surgeon and fighting the medical system that shackles so many doctors. It was a reality I'd struggled with until 2021, when I finally hit my breaking point. I was up until midnight finishing patient notes after seeing 40 patients in a single day — a routine that was all too common — when I stumbled on a webinar hosted by Matt Gillogly while catching up on my hundreds of emails. In the webinar, Gillogly, a business coach, spoke about how there were ways to escape the clutches of the failing insurance-based healthcare system. As I listened, it felt like he was speaking directly to me.

So, this tired, burned-out, overworked, and undercompensated orthopedic surgeon with the weight of insurance companies and the medical system on his back signed up to receive a copy of Gillogly's book, *The Anatomy of a 7-Figure Medical Practice.* His words cracked open a door I didn't know existed and showed me a way out of the insurance trap — a way back to the joy of medicine.

That book planted the seed for the one you're reading now.

Piece by piece, God's plan revealed itself. A chance email at midnight. A bar seat next to Nicole. Books by Michael and Ed that reshaped my thinking. Countless hours writing, revising, and pushing through fear.

Eventually, the manuscript was finished, and I held the book I once thought impossible to write.

Now I can say without hesitation that this book exists because of God's hand and because of the people He placed in my path.

I thank God first.

I thank Ed Rush for teaching me how to truly hear His voice.

I thank Nicole Gebhardt for showing up that night in Las Vegas and walking with me every step of this journey. Nicole, you, Kim, Kimberly, Tami, Ellen, and your whole team are the best! And reader, if you're thinking of writing a book, contact Nicole.

I thank Michael Hauge for the endless hours spent helping me shape my stories. I so enjoyed working with you and consider you a dear and trusted friend. Similarly, if you are writing a book, investing in working with Michael Hauge will be some of the best dollars you ever spend... and you'll have a lot of fun too.

I thank Russell Brunson and Coach Vince for making the connection with Nicole possible.

And I thank Matt Gillogly, whose book gave me the courage to break free from the chains of the insurance system, who strongly encouraged me to write my own book, and who was the spark and catalyst for going *all in* on Knee Repair, NOT Knee Replacement and regenerative, non-insurance-based medicine resulting in true freedom for me, my staff, and especially our patients!

I'm still a little scared of how people will respond to this book, but I'm also proud of this work and deeply grateful for the experience. My hope is that this book will help patients find a path toward healing beyond replacement surgery, inspire doctors to reclaim their joy, and rally all of us toward the mission of ending the need for knee replacements by 2043.

Thank you for joining me in this movement. Together, we can make the vision real. #KneeReplacementFreeBy43.

# ACKNOWLEDGMENTS

First and foremost, I thank God. In the human world, I first thank my wife, Cristina, for being the most supportive, loving, and amazing life partner anyone could hope for. Thank you for sticking with me through thick and thin and through all of my crazy journeys! Your encouragement and strength have carried me through this process.

I thank my children: Alexandra, your loving and supportive husband, Kevin, and the star of this book, my granddaughter, Lyla Bella; Marc Jr., your wonderful wife, Hannah, and my beautiful baby granddaughter, Pia; and my youngest, "Daddy's little girl," Isabella.

I thank my mother and father (and my grandparents, aunts, uncles, brother, three sisters, brothers-in-law, sister-in-law, cousins, as well as the next generation of nieces and nephews) for showing me that faith, family, and hard work are not always easy, but they do always pay off.

To all my patients — especially those who are part of this book — and the countless others who have trusted me and my team: thank you. I thank all my future patients who, as a result of this book, will also place their trust in me, my team, and my Victory Method for Functional & Musculoskeletal Restoration.

And speaking of my team, I especially thank our current team of Addison, Allison, Cristina, Jamie, Jessica, Jordan, Kayci, Luciano, and Stephanie. You have all been truly supportive, and I am grateful for the times when you covered for me on all the days I had to work from home while writing this. You are **ALL IN**, and I will always appreciate that.

Thank you to all the past team members of Victory Sports Medicine & Orthopedics and Victory In Motion. You have all, in your own way, helped shape and write a part of this book, and I will never forget that.

# DR. PIETROPAOLI

Dr. Marc Pietropaoli is a fellowship-trained sports medicine orthopedic surgeon, regenerative medicine expert, and founder of Victory In Motion, home of Knee Repair, NOT Knee Replacement. Since 1998, he has dedicated his career to pioneering alternatives to invasive joint replacement surgery.

Trained under world-renowned sports medicine surgeons Dr. James R. Andrews and Dr. William G. Clancy, Dr. Pietropaoli was among the earliest physicians in the United States to integrate regenerative treatments like bone marrow aspirate cells and platelet-rich plasma into orthopedic care.

In October 2021, he became the first surgeon in the world to perform an FDA-indicated Bridge-Enhanced ACL Restoration procedure outside of clinical trials, an achievement that led to his work being formally recognized on the floor of the United States Congress and entered into the Congressional Record by Representative John Katko on December 24, 2021.

His innovative programs blend advanced biologics, precision diagnostics, cutting-edge laser therapy, total-body fitness, genetic-based nutrition, and functional and holistic recovery, and have helped thousands of people avoid unnecessary knee and other joint replacements. These outcomes are tracked through the DataBiologics national registry, where his results consistently rank among the best in the country.

His mission is bold but clear: to end the need for knee replacement surgeries worldwide by the year 2043 — a vision he calls Knee Replacement Free by '43.

At the heart of this mission are faith, family, and hard work — values Dr. Pietropaoli learned from his parents and grandparents. These principles not only shaped his upbringing but also continue to drive his relentless pursuit of better solutions for patients who are told they have no other option.

Outside the clinic, Dr. Pietropaoli is devoted to his wife, Cristina, their children, and grandchildren. Also known as #FunFarmerDrP, he enjoys running marathons, working in his garden, tapping maple trees for syrup, and making limoncello from homegrown lemons with his father-in-law. He believes the same principles that make soil fertile — care, patience, and resiliency — are the ones that help people flourish in both medicine and life.

## GET IN TOUCH

Contact:      info@VictoryInMotion.com
Website:      VictoryInMotion.com

## SOCIAL

Facebook:     @victoryinmotion1
Instagram:    @victoryinmotion1 and @drmarcpietropaoli
TikTok:       @victoryinmotion1 and @drmarcpietropaoli
YouTube:      @victoryinmotion1
LinkedIn:     Marc Pietropaoli, MD

# READY TO SCHEDULE YOUR CLARITY DAY?

If you're ready to take the next step in your healing journey and schedule your Clarity Day, here's how to get started:

- Call our office: 315-993-KNEE
- Visit our website: www.victoryinmotion.com
- Scan the QR code below for immediate scheduling

Schedule Your Clarity Day HERE

**Krnkr.com/c-d-e-order-form**

www.ingramcontent.com/pod-product-compliance
Lightning Source LLC
Chambersburg PA
CBHW060231030426
42335CB00014B/1410